P9-AGM-595

LICK THE SUGAR HABIT

Nancy Appleton, Ph.D.

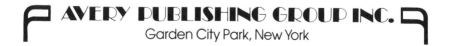
AVERY PUBLISHING GROUP INC.
Garden City Park, New York

The information in this book is not intended as medical advice. Its intention is solely informational and educational. It is assumed that the reader will consult a medical or health professional should the need for one be warranted.

NANCY APPLETON earned her Ph.D. in Nutrition and is a nutritional consultant, researcher, author, and speaker. She shares in this book the self-help program that made her well after a lifetime addiction to sugar. "Since childhood I was subject to illness, including allergies, boils, candida, a calcium deposit removed from my chest, chronic bronchitis, and numerous bouts of pneumonia," she explains. "Only when I changed my diet and life-style was I able to reverse the degenerative process and return my body to health." Nancy Appleton is also the author of *Healthy Bones: What You Should Know About Osteoporosis.*

Copyright © 1988 by Nancy Appleton

ISBN 0-89529-386-2

Printed in the United States of America by Paragon Press, Honesdale, PA.

10 9

Contents

INTRODUCTION BY LENDON SMITH, M.D., vii

FOREWORD BY SHIRLEY LORENZANI, PH.D., ix

PREFACE BY BRUCE PACETTI, D.D.S., xi

A PERSONAL WORD FROM THE AUTHOR, xiii

1. **I WAS A SUGARHOLIC,** 1
   A Twist of Fate, 3
   Are You a Sugarholic? 5
   How You Feel Is up to You, 7
   Sugar—the Sour Facts, 8

2. **SUGAR'S UNBALANCING ACT,** 12
   Page's Research, 13
   Mineral Relationships, 15
   Endocrine Glands, 17
   Enzymes, 19

3. **ALL ABOUT ALLERGIES,** 21
   What's Ahead? 28

4. **THE DESTRUCTION OF THE IMMUNE SYSTEM,** 30
   Stage I: Acute Reaction, 32
   Stage II: Chronic Reaction, 33
   Stage III: Degenerative Reaction, 36
   Some Other Studies, 37

5. **THE CONSEQUENCES,** 41
   Hypoglycemia, 42
   Diabetes, 44
   Constipation, 46
   Stomach or Intestinal Gas, 48
   Arthritis, 49

Asthma, 51
Headaches, 52
Psoriasis, 53
Cancer, 54
Osteoporosis, 56
Heart Disease, 62
Obesity, 65
Candida Albicans, 67
Tooth Decay, 68
Multiple Sclerosis, 71
Inflammatory Bowel Disease, 71
Canker Sores, 73
Gallstones, 73
Cystic Fibrosis, 74
Future Generations, 75

6. SUGAR'S HELPERS, 78
Alcohol, 78
Caffeine, 81
Drugs, 83
Rancid Fats, 86
Other Overcooked Foods, 87
Aspirin, 89
Food Additives, 91
Sweeteners, 93
Mercury, 95

7. STRESS, 97
Psychological Stress, 98
Sugar and Psychological Stress, 99
How to Handle Stress, 101

8. A PRACTICAL LIFE PLAN FOR ATTAINING AND
MAINTAINING GOOD HEALTH, 103
Four Arenas, 105
A Test to Determine Homeostasis in Your Body, 109
Food Plans, 110
Food Categories, 112
Simple Suggestions for Breakfasts and Snacks, 116
Health-Promoting Eating Habits, 117

9. SELF-HELP TECHNIQUES, 118

10. EPILOGUE, 124
RECIPES, 126
GLOSSARY, 138
BIBLIOGRAPHY, 145
INDEX, 159
BODY CHEMISTRY TEST KIT ORDER FORM, 162

Introduction

We have heard of the evils of sugar from every writer in the world, except, of course, from the sugar industry. So what right does Nancy Appleton have to write a book that is going to tell us to stop eating sugar? We've heard that old saw before. But wait, gentle reader! There is something in this book of which you are not aware—good and compelling reasons to avoid the sweet stuff.

The biochemical pathway from ingestion to enzyme function decay is traced in such a clear, understandable way that the most confirmed sugarholic will at least cut down on the intake a smidge. How sugar affects the calcium/phosphorus ratio in the bloodstream, how this seems to be the common pathway of stress, and how this stress can lead to degenerative disease are described and documented. I would get a headache, someone else would get migraine, colitis, asthma, eczema, or depression. A method for self-testing at home and monitoring the nutritional treatment is also presented.

Nancy Appleton's own addiction and recovery give her story a unique viewpoint. She documents the problems stemming from too much sugar and gives self-help techniques and recipes to lick the sugar habit.

A strong case is made for each of us to take responsibility for our own health. Appleton makes it clear that we are responsible for what we eat, think, do, and say. We are not victims of the twentieth-century life-style, but many of us do choose a life-style that leads to the degenerative disease process.

I recommend this book to everyone who has made personal health a priority, and every person who wants to remove sugar from her or his diet. For sugarholics *Lick the Sugar Habit* is an absolute must.

Lendon Smith, M.D.

Foreword

On what do we place the blame for the poor health of modern man? Diet is surely a major factor.

Eggs, that's it. Quick, everyone! Switch to sweet rolls and coffee before the eggs clog your arteries! On, no—it's the fat. No more red meat, cut out the butter, watch out for the deadly salad dressing! No, no—salt is the villain. Go for bland, hide the shaker!

Have you noticed that few experts mention sugar? Pure and white, it innocently makes its way into much of our food and into our mouths. If it's so-o-o-o-o-o good, how could it be so bad? Who would not want to believe that it's the omelet rather than the ice cream that's doing us in? Apple pie and ice cream is, after all, the national dish.

Lick the Sugar Habit suggests that sugar eating, our national pastime, is linked to disease, our leading growth industry. We've heard this theory before. Never before, however, has it been presented so clearly and without fanaticism. Nancy Appleton is not saying that sugar is the only cause of disease. She is saying that sugar is a major contributor to the disease process. She presents sugar as one of the stress factors that weaken our defenses against illness.

Sounds reasonable, doesn't it? Eliminating sugar from

the diet is also reasonable. Have you ever cut out sugar? That's when life can get very unreasonable. Cold-turkey withdrawal from sugar can bring on the shakes, fever, depression, and headaches. At that point it seems more reasonable to continue the addiction.

Lick the Sugar Habit is a lifesaver, literally. It is a guide to getting unhooked from sugar. Tips on shopping, snacking, supportive friendships, and exercise make this book much more than another synopsis of all the studies on diet and disease.

Even more appealing, Nancy Appleton has been there. Once a sugarholic, she has won the battle against sugar addiction and has been rewarded with vibrant health. The empathy she brings to this subject is genuine. She knows the detrimental effects of sugar.

Are you ready for renewed health and vitality? Will you make the effort to heal and prevent heart disease, cancer, diabetes, arthritis, and osteoporosis?

The most important effort, for many of us, is licking the sugar habit. Unless that is done, all else may be largely wasted effort. The beneficial effects of exercise are lessened by a sugar diet. The roller-coaster emotions of a sugarholic often wreck supportive relationships. A sugar-dependent person is often too tired to function well at home or at work.

If you are ready to be the best that you can be, this book is for you. Sugar-free may be the missing piece in your puzzle for health.

Shirley Lorenzani, Ph.D.

Preface

Nancy Appleton relates her personal story, and with clear scientific analysis gives an understanding of how disease originates and what one can do about it. She also tells how one can improve and monitor one's basic health, and how one can enhance the response to any necessary doctoring.

I have spent the last fifteen years of my professional life doing research, clinically applying and lecturing on an obscure biological principle, which is showing evidence of being the common denominator of all disease. It was like a breath of fresh air for me to see how easily Nancy Appleton understood the Body Chemistry Principle the first time I met and exchanged ideas with her. The Body Chemistry Principle is usually not easily understood by health care practitioners.

The Body Chemistry Principle has to do with the functioning of the body systems which depend upon the body's chemical balances. These systems include the immune system, endocrine system, and digestive system, among others.

Several civilizations have crumbled because of a lack of knowledge about the Body Chemistry Principle. Our civilization is now showing the first signs. Insurance companies are concerned today because statistics show that by

1990, 75 percent of our adult population will have a degenerative disease.

Few Americans today die of old age. Instead, heart attacks, strokes, cancer, and diabetes are the usual causes of death. Arthritis, indigestion, influenza, and constipation are also a normal part of our lives. In the future, will coronary bypasses, artificial hearts and kidneys, hysterectomies, reading glasses, PMS, false teeth, and plastic hip joints be accepted also? They need not be. As always, the fittest will survive and live. The fittest now will be those who understand the Body Chemistry Principle. Appleton's book is a practical introduction to this most vital subject.

Bruce Pacetti, D.D.S.

A Personal Word from the Author

I would like to take this opportunity to recognize a special debt of gratitude to Bruce Pacetti, D.D.S.

His knowledge of the Body Chemistry Principle along with the willingness with which he communicated it to me as well as to others is the bedrock foundation of my successful effort to regain my health.

Many of my ideas in this book come from our many talks and his lectures. Not only did I regain my health, but through his understanding and love, a special friendship has developed.

Nancy Appleton, Ph.D.

1 | I Was a Sugarholic

When I was a child, a bakery truck used to come regularly to the back door of our house. If my mother wasn't around, I could buy anything I wanted and charge it—no one seemed to know who had charged what when the bakery bill came. I would buy six doughnuts, four nut bars, and a couple of coffee cakes, hide them from the rest of the family, and eat them in private. In two days all of the goodies would be gone, and I'd wait for the bakery truck and more sweet morsels.

Although I didn't realize it, I was a sugarholic and a chocoholic. Almost from birth I craved the stuff. In my early childhood I was plagued with bothersome allergies—the signals of an unbalanced body chemistry. My nose ran continually, and so did my eyes. I was constantly sticking fingers in my ears to try to stop the itching, rubbing my fingers over my throat or even scratching the back of my throat with my tongue for the same reason. Like most people, I misread these body signals and continued my dangerous dietary habits.

My upsetting addiction became worse in my teenage

years. I played tennis for four hours a day, every day, and the calories I burned up on the tennis court more than compensated for the calories in the sweets I continued to eat. Therefore, I could consume an incredible amount of sugar and chocolate and not gain weight, even though I was upsetting my body chemistry. After winning a tennis tournament, I would treat myself to two hot-fudge sundaes. When I would lose a tournament, I would eat a whole package of chocolate cookies. Winner or loser, I was a loser. Again, I just wasn't aware of the connection between my sweet addiction, upset body chemistry, and illness.

All I knew at that age was that I wasn't fat—just young, strong, and unhealthy. Every tooth in my mouth was eventually filled with gold or silver. My first bout with pneumonia came at age thirteen, and it put me in the hospital for two weeks. During my second year in college I had a large tumor removed from my chest, which, after a great deal of expensive investigation, turned out to be nothing but a calcium deposit. No one told me that my body was unable to digest milk and calcium properly; no one suggested that the sugar in my diet and other life-style factors might be upsetting my body chemistry and causing my increasing health problems. I continued to ignore the signals my body was giving me and, in my ignorance, went right on with my unhealthy life-style.

I spent my junior year of college studying in Switzerland, land of chocolate. While in Geneva, I phoned a nearby chocolate factory, explained that I was a food and nutrition major, and asked for a tour. What I really wanted, of course, were the chocolate samples at the end of the line. That little trip fed my habit for about a week. This time, the weight game didn't work. Because I was traveling and not playing my usual four hours of tennis every day, I wasn't burning off the excess calories. I came back from Europe thirty pounds overweight, my sugar and chocolate cravings stronger than ever.

My adult life was plagued with boils, canker sores,

varicose veins, headaches, constipation, fatigue, colds, flu, and four more bouts with pneumonia—the results of a life-style which promoted an upset body chemistry. Each time I became sick with pneumonia, recovery took longer; my immune system was being continually weakened by my dietary habits and my life-style. After my last pneumonia, my cough lasted for six months. Every specialist I consulted diagnosed my problem as chronic bronchitis. "Take antibiotics ten days out of the month for the rest of your life," I was told over and over. Not one doctor said, "What do you put in your mouth, what do you eat?"

I was forty years old, and would soon find that I knew little about nutrition, sugar, allergies, or health. Yet although I still believed that doctors would take care of me, somehow I just couldn't swallow their diagnoses any easier than I could swallow antibiotics ten days a month for the rest of my life. As my cough continued, I decided to try yoga. I thought that if I stood on my head long enough, the phlegm would come out of my chest. Wrong again. My cough was still there after hours of viewing the world upside down. I didn't yet know that an upset body will produce excess phlegm right side up or upside down.

A Twist of Fate

A friend suggested that if I wanted to explore some different ideas on health, the book section of a health food store would be a good place to look. This idea appealed to the book lover in me, and I soon encountered *The Pulse Test*, by Arthur F. Coca, M.D. This book said it was possible to detect food allergies by comparing one's pulse before eating the food in question and after. If my pulse increased ten to twelve beats per minute after I ate the food,

Coca suggested, I was not metabolizing that food correctly, and was allergic to it.

Being a good do-it-yourselfer, I took my pulse after awakening and found that I had a resting pulse rate of sixty beats per minute. Remembering that as a child I had suffered from stomach cramps, gas, and allergies after eating ice cream, I drank one glass of milk and took my pulse shortly after. I couldn't believe it—my pulse had jumped from sixty beats to eighty in just a few minutes. I repeated the experiment the next morning, with the same results.*

That was eight years ago, and it was the beginning of a new life. I began seeing many different types of clinicians: homeopathic doctors, naturopaths, orthomolecular doctors, and clinical ecologists. These doctors deal with a variety of methods for healing the body other than antibiotics and surgery. They changed my diet, gave me supplements, and offered homeopathic medicines that might heal my body. It took me a long time to realize that there is no magic pill and that even a lot of pills together do not make a magic potion. The pills would help to some degree, but as long as I was feeding my body abusive foods and continually upsetting my body chemistry, all the pills in the world would not help. It's like continuously tapping one's head with a small hammer and wondering why aspirin isn't getting rid of the headache!

Awareness and change take time, and so does healing. There is no such thing as instant health, and the damage I had done to my body over the course of forty years would not be undone overnight. The more I became in touch with my body, the easier it was to discover what it did and didn't need. My body was so out of homeostasis (balance) that it was giving me confusing signals because often the foods that

---

*I must warn you that not all foods to which you've developed allergies alter your pulse. But after ingesting a food, if your pulse rate increases or decreases at least ten beats per minute over the resting rate, the odds are great that you are not metabolizing the food correctly. You have developed an allergic sensitivity to it.

satisfy a craving also deepen the addiction and upset. Getting in touch with my allergies, cravings, addictions, headaches, sneezes and wheezes was a slow, painful process, but it was enlightening. Although I often had to backtrack, I eventually learned about myself and what it meant to feel well.

Are You a Sugarholic?

What signals is your body giving you? Are you a sugarholic? This quiz will help you determine how pervasive refined sugar is in your life-style, and what effect it's having on your body. Refined sugar includes sucrose, honey, fructose, glucose, dextrose, levulose, maltose, raw sugar, turbinato sugar, maple sugar, galactose, brown sugar, invert sugar, dextrine, barley malt, rice syrup, corn sweetener, and corn syrup. All of these are simple sugars. They take very little time to digest and get into the bloodstream, where they perform the same disturbance to your body chemistry as table sugar. These substances are found in doughnuts, processed foods, jelly on your toast, ice cream, candy bars, packaged cereal, soft drinks, catsup, beer, chewing tobacco, chewing gum, and any product which lists sugar among its ingredients. Answer each question as truthfully as you can; you're not going to be graded, and no one is looking over your shoulder. Be honest with yourself—your health depends on it.

	TRUE	FALSE
1. I don't eat refined sugar every day.	_____	_____
2. I can go for more than a day without eating some type of sugar-containing food.	_____	_____

	TRUE	FALSE
3. I never have cravings for sugar, coffee, chocolate, peanut butter, or alcohol.	_____	_____
4. I've never hidden candy or other sweets around my home in order to find and eat them later.	_____	_____
5. I can stop after one piece of candy or one bite of pastry.	_____	_____
6. There are times when I have no sugar of any kind in my home.	_____	_____
7. I can go for three or more hours without eating and not experience the shakes, fatigue, perspiration, irritability, depressions, or anxiety.	_____	_____
8. I can have candy and other sweets in my home and not eat them.	_____	_____
9. I don't eat something sweet after every meal.	_____	_____
10. I rarely drink coffee and eat doughnuts or sweet rolls for breakfast.	_____	_____
11. I can go for more than an hour after waking up in the morning without eating.	_____	_____
12. I can go from one day to the next without drinking a soft drink.	_____	_____

If you answered "false" to more than four of these statements, chances are that you are sugar-sensitive. You probably are allergic to sugar, and probably also addicted to it—the same way an alcoholic is addicted to alcohol. You crave sugar, have withdrawal symptoms when you don't get it, and probably feel better for a short time after you've eaten it. In eating sugar to feel better, you are actually making your condition worse.

If you answered "false" to four questions or fewer, that doesn't prove you don't have a problem with sugar. Perhaps you aren't addicted to it, but perhaps you don't quite realize just how much sugar you're eating. According to the United States Department of Agriculture, the average American consumes more than 130 pounds of sugar and sweeteners a year, most of it hidden or contained in other foods (96 percent of cranberry sauce's calories and 63 percent of catsup's calories are sugar). We eat over 10 pounds of sugar each month, nearly 4½ cups per week or 30 to 33 teaspoonfuls of sugar every day. That's over 20 percent of our daily caloric intake spent on a refined food which upsets body chemistry and has no nutritional value, since refined sugar is 99.4 to 99.7 percent pure calories—no vitamins, minerals, or proteins, just simple carbohydrates.

How You Feel Is up to You

My experience is a classic example of what I've called the "degenerative disease process." All my ailments were caused by the substances I put into my body. The excess sugar that I ate so obsessively led to a disturbance of mineral relationships in my system—leading to a calcium excess so severe that it built up in my chest. This mineral imbalance made my enzymes (those chemicals in the body that help digest food) incapable of digesting food properly, and I developed classic allergic symptoms due to the undigested food. My immune system wore itself down reacting to these toxic foods, and I became extremely susceptible to disease.

The process that started with the excess consumption of

sugar ended in tooth decay, pneumonia, and bronchitis. It was mainly when I removed sugar from my diet that my body was able to regain health. I realized then, for the first time, that if I stopped doing to my body what I had done to make it sick, my body would heal itself.

Having shared my health saga with many people, I know now that many of us go through life not knowing what it is to feel well. We are somewhere between health and disease most of the time, our symptoms and body signals oscillating between not-so-bad and miserable. Since that is all we know, we start believing this is how everyone feels.

Still, it is possible to feel better—and if you really want to, chances are that you can. *It is up to you.* You can make yourself sick by ingesting harmful substances or, by becoming aware of what serves your health and listening to your body's signals, you can stop upsetting the body and let the body heal itself.

If, on the other hand, you ignore the signals your body is sending, you force doctors to use stronger and more dangerous techniques, and relegate yourself to the victim role. Doctors are accustomed to treating conditions that have progressed to a point that there are serious complaints (severe pain, heart palpitations, swollen joints, or rapid weight loss). They see these drastic conditions and they take drastic measures.

Sugar—the Sour Facts

Now, I don't eat any sugar, and I know many others who don't, so many of you must be getting more than 130 pounds. We humans need only two teaspoons of sugar in our body at any time in order to function properly. This amount can be obtained easily through the digestion of carbohydrates, protein, and fats. Even if we were to eat no glucose or refined sugar at all, our bodies would still have plenty of sugar. Every extra teaspoon of refined sugar you eat works to throw the body out of balance and compromise its health.

Ironically the initial damage done by excess sugar makes it that much harder to give up. Refined sugar is made up of two simple sugars, glucose and fructose. When a person eats sugar continually, the body becomes inefficient at manufacturing glucose from complex carbohydrates, protein, and fats. The mechanisms in the body which perform this task shut down from disuse, causing the blood glucose level to drop. The cravings, perspiration, shakes, and depression that follow send the sugarholic running for the nearest candy bar or cookie jar, and the vicious cycle continues. These sweets may bring the blood sugar back to normal for the moment, but the body chemistry is being upset. When the individual gets to a point where body chemistry cannot rebalance, health breakdowns result.

Refined sugar, as tempting as it may be in all those cakes, candies, and cups of coffee, is, in fact, more of a drugging pharmaceutical chemical than it is a nurturing food. It has been stripped of all its nutrients and robs the body of nutrients during the process of digestion and metabolism. The minerals needed to digest sugar—chromium, manganese, cobalt, copper, zinc, and magnesium—have been stripped away in the refining process, and the body has to deplete its own mineral reserves to use the refined sugar.

Glucose, as high in calories as refined sugar, is in effect a predigested food that undergoes no processing at all in the stomach or intestines. Yet there is no law requiring that glucose be listed with other ingredients on the label of any package! The food industry uses glucose as a cheap filler; since it is not as sweet as sugar and therefore unrecognizable, many people consume large quantities of glucose without realizing it. If you eat packaged foods such as cereal, bakery goods, sauces, and processed meats, chances are you're getting more sugar than you bargained for—maybe 130 pounds more!

This high consumption wasn't always the case. It's only in the last two centuries that sugar has become a staple of American diets. In colonial America table sugar cost $2.40 a pound, as opposed to $.35 a pound today. Sugar was an expensive luxury then, and a cube of sugar in a Christmas stocking was considered a real treat. In 1795 a large-scale method of granulating sugar was devised, and Louisiana farmers began growing sugarcane as a major crop. Sugar prices went down, availability went up, and Americans began eating too much of it.

Human evolution has not yet caught up with the sugar industry. For many thousands of years, mankind ate no sugar at all. Prehistoric man ate basically raw meat; later, seeds and nuts were added to the diet, and with the birth of agriculture came vegetables, legumes, and fruits. Two hundred years of sugar is merely a moment compared to this, and we have not evolved with mechanisms to cope with this glut. Therefore, our bodies are unable to metabolize such large amounts of sugar on a daily basis. In compensating for the excess, our organs and glands become overworked, exhausted, and eventually they malfunction. This is what we know as degenerative disease.

If you're a sugarholic, as I was, your body is telling you quite bluntly that sugar is causing problems. Addiction is closely related to allergy; the body has become so accustomed to compensating for the presence of the allergenic substance that when the substance is removed, withdrawal symptoms occur. Your sugar cravings are a direct indication that sugar is at work destroying your immune system.

There are many other ways in which a sugar problem can manifest itself. You may become allergic to other foods (see Chapter 3). You may experience headaches, joint pains, gas pains, bloating, fatigue, and other ailments which are not as easily traced to sugar. For this reason, many who are not sugarholics, who do not feel cravings for sugar or indulge their sweet tooth, refuse to believe that sugar is the cause of their problems. They continue their dietary indiscretions, and the disease process is allowed to advance.

Therefore, it's important to understand exactly how sugar, even a little sugar, starts this chain reaction. The pages that follow represent a step-by-step journey down this pathway to degenerative disease. You'll learn how sugar throws the body out of balance and causes food allergies, endocrine problems, hypoglycemia, diabetes, tooth decay, osteoporosis, arthritis, cancer, and all degenerative diseases. You'll discover ways to rid yourself of these problems by removing sugar and other harmful substances from your diet. You'll also find concrete self-help techniques for doing just that. These ideas can lead you to a philosophy of responsibility instead of a philosophy of helplessness in matters of health. When we know we've created ill health, we can choose to stop it.

2 | Sugar's Unbalancing Act

Minerals are essential to many bodily functions. They give rigidity to the hard tissues of the body, the bones and teeth. Minerals also help to maintain a balance in the blood and body tissues between acidity and alkalinity. Some minerals have specific functions in the transmission of nerve impulses throughout the body; others are important in the process of digestion.

Those minerals that are highly essential to the body include: calcium and phosphorus, which, in addition to building strong bones, activate enzymes needed for important metabolic functions; magnesium, which is also both a structural material and an enzyme catalyst; iron, which contributes to enzymes as well as being an important part of the blood's hemoglobin; iodine, which is necessary to the proper functioning of the thyroid gland; and zinc, without which the enzyme alcohol dehydrogenase cannot perform its function of oxidizing alcohol in the liver.

The average person consumes 20 percent of his or her calories from some form of refined sugar. This makes it difficult for the body to get the nutrients it needs from the other 80 percent. Many people think that they can eat anything they want as long as they take their multivitamin and mineral pill daily. Sugar so upsets the body chemistry that it doesn't matter what else you put in your mouth; neither healthful food nor junk food will digest properly.

Somewhere along the path of creating health for myself, I realized how important it was to have enough of the right vitamins, minerals, essential fatty acids, and amino acids in my diet. Therefore, I became very aware of having a diet that included all those nutrients. I would sit down to a meal with all the nutrients in it. Then, because I had been so good with my perfect nutrient-filled meal, I would treat myself to a piece of chocolate cake—negating many positive effects the nutrients might have had.

Many people in the nutrition field have not come to the understanding that as long as sugar is eaten, nutrients will be unavailable to the body. The required daily allowance (RDA) of vitamins and minerals set up by the government is not a valid measure for health; many people do meet those requirements through food or supplements, but because sugar changes their body chemistry, the cells can't fully benefit from those vitamins and minerals.

Page's Research

The disastrous effect of sugar on the calcium/phosphorus ratio was first discovered by Dr. Melvin Page, a dentist who noted bone loss in his patients, which he understood as calcium deficiency. Yet these patients all showed normal calcium in their blood. Page consulted with several physicians as to how this could be, and the answer was always the same: "If there are ten units of calcium in the blood, then there is enough calcium in the body." What they didn't realize—and many still don't—is that minerals work only in relation to each other.

Fortunately Page could not accept their explanation. He started looking at other minerals in the body. He found that if he could get a patient's calcium/phosphorus ratio to be the optimum 10 to 4, the symptoms that led to tooth decay and bone loss, as well as many other negative symptoms, would simply go away. Through further investigation, he discovered that sugar caused the phosphorus to decrease and the calcium to increase. Therefore, although there was more than the necessary amount of calcium in the body, less of it could be used because of the drop in phosphorus. Once he took his patients off sugar and put them on a diet of whole foods, their dental problems would disappear and so would many other problems.

Researchers have since found that ingesting sugar increases the rate at which we excrete calcium. If, when we eat sugar, our blood calcium goes up and we also excrete it, we must be pulling it from the bones and tissues because that is the only place it is stored in the body. Calcium depletion of the bones makes them fragile and causes osteoporosis. Often a doctor will recommend taking extra calcium to combat this calcium depletion, but this calcium can become toxic if the other minerals are not in balance with it. It would be far better to cut sugar out of the diet; in most cases, it is sugar which is throwing the minerals out of balance and causing the calcium deficiency in the first place.

Every time we ingest even two teaspoons of sugar, the mineral ratios in our bodies can change. The vitamins and minerals in our bodies are always changing—that is what homeostasis involves, a continual fine-tuning of the body chemistry. Sugar can cause these micronutrients to change radically, throwing the blood chemistry out of homeostasis. Some minerals increase, some decrease, and delicate ratios are disturbed. In healthy people the minerals come back into relationship soon; in sick people the minerals stay out of relationship for hours, and sometimes they do not come back at all. When minerals are out of balance day after day, year after year, and possibly through generations, the ability of the body to balance back into homeostasis is exhausted. The body no longer can fine-tune itself.

Mineral Relationships

Minerals work only in relation to one another. If one of the minerals is deficient in the body, others don't function as well. Conversely, when one mineral increases and another does not, the mineral that has increased becomes toxic because it is no longer in correct ratio or mineral relationship with the one that has not increased. That's why some vitamins and minerals are prescribed only in conjunction with certain others. It's like trying to make French toast with a whole loaf of bread and only one egg; you may have the right ingredients, but you won't get French toast.

Other researchers have found the same evidence. Dr. Boy Frame and Dr. Geoffrey Marel found that "recent experimental evidence in the nutrition of trace elements suggests that a variety of imbalances in trace metal concentrations may have more importance than an abnormal concentration of any single trace element."

This interrelationship of minerals, and the damage that can be caused by disturbing it, can readily be seen in the case of calcium and phosphorus, two of the most important minerals in the body. The normal ratio of these minerals is 10 units of calcium to 4 units of phosphorus, or 2.5 times as much calcium as phosphorus. Since minerals work properly only when they are in the correct ratio, when the phosphorus decreases, the functioning calcium decreases. If there are only 2 units of phosphorus, then only 2.5 times that, or 5

FIGURE 2-1

MINERAL WHEEL

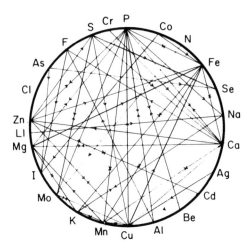

Dr. Paul Eck
Analytical Research Labs, Inc.
Phoenix, Arizona

units of calcium, will be functioning; the rest of the calcium will become harmful. On the other hand, if calcium increases to 12, but the phosphorus remains at 4, then the extra 2 units of calcium will become toxic.

If only 5 units of calcium are functioning, then the body is getting only half of the calcium it needs, since the optimum amount is 10. Therefore, it is possible to have both toxic calcium and a calcium deficiency in the body at the same time, a seeming contradiction. Toxic or nonfunctioning calcium can cause kidney stones, arthritis, hardening of the arteries, cataracts, and plaque on the teeth. In my case, toxic calcium had been accumulating in my body since birth, and eventually resulted in the calcium deposit which was removed from my chest.

Endocrine Glands

Your own endocrine glandular system determines which minerals are going to be the most affected by sugar. This system of glands is the automatic pilot of the processes in our body; it regulates all involuntary or unconscious activities. Respiration, heartbeat, digestion and assimilation of food, elimination, body temperature, physical integrity, equilibrium, and balanced body chemistry—all come under the supervision of one or more of the endocrine glands.

These endocrine glands include the pancreas, the pituitary, the thyroid and hypothalamus, the adrenals, and the gonads. Each gland sends hormones into the bloodstream, chemical messengers which determine how the body works. The intake of harmful foods like sugar reduces the efficiency of the glands, causing a smaller secretion or an altered composition of hormones. This, in turn, has a detrimental effect on the body chemistry.

Each of us has inherited some weak glands and some strong glands. If our body stays in balance because of a healthy life-style, neither the weak nor the strong glands will hurt us. If we destroy our body chemistry through dietary indiscretions, our weak glands will become exhausted and our strong glands, in compensating for the weak ones, will become exhausted as well.

The endocrine system is designed so that each gland has an opposite in terms of these strengths and weaknesses; corresponding glands are indicated in Figure 2-2. If you have a genetic potential to be, say, a 6 out of a possible 10 rating in the thyroid, then the pancreas will be a 10. When your body chemistry becomes unbalanced, the pancreas may overcompensate and go up to a 12. Since the function of the pancreas is to secrete insulin, sodium bicarbonate, and pancreatic enzymes, an excess of these substances may occur. If you were also born with a weak anterior pituitary, the pancreas would have to work even harder to compensate.

FIGURE 2-2

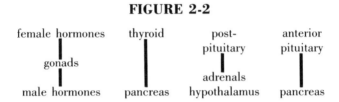

Each person's inherited endocrine system produces individual psychological and physical characteristics. A person with a hyperthyroid, whose chemistry is routinely upset, will suffer from heavy perspiration, emotional ups and downs, and hyperenergy. People with a weak postpituitary tend to become extremely emotional. If they go to a sad movie and their body chemistries are in balance, they will cry. If they go to a sad movie, eat chocolate, and drink soft drinks, which upsets their body chemistries, they will become devastated, even hysterical.

This was the case with me. I was born with a potential toward a weak postpituitary and anterior pituitary, in addition to a weak thyroid. I remember many a time going to a movie as a child and crying my heart out. Everyone around me thought I was crazy. One time, after seeing a movie called *No Sad Songs for Me* (about a mother of two young children who was dying of cancer and maneuvering her husband to fall in love with his secretary so he would have someone after she died), I cried through half the movie, all the way home, and even cried myself to sleep. Of course, the sugar that I was eating so obsessively had thrown my chemistry into disarray and was causing my extreme reactions.

When a person ingests sugar, certain glands are accelerated to function at more than normal speed. These include the pancreas, which secretes the insulin needed to metabolize sugar, and a part of the adrenal gland called the adrenal medulla, which produces epinephrine (adrenaline), a hormone responsible for stimulating the breakdown of stored glycogen back to usable glucose. These glands also control the assimilation of calcium; the faster they work, the more calcium is absorbed into the blood, resulting in the calcium/phosphorus imbalance discussed earlier.

Other glands, such as the thyroid and the adrenals, are reduced by sugar in their action to less than a normal level. These are the glands which control the assimilation of phosphorus; just as the overstimulation of the calcium regulators causes an increase in calcium, the suppression of these phosphorus regulators leads to a decrease in phosphorus. Such a decrease, as we have seen, means a decrease in usable calcium, even as the overall calcium level in the blood rises. The vicious cycle continues.

The levels of calcium and phosphorus in the blood indicate whether the endocrine system is in balance or not. Since the endocrines are those glands that determine metabolism, it is obvious that their balance or lack of balance will result in the health or lack or health of the individual. Metabolism is the process by which food is broken down into essential nutrients which can be absorbed by the cells of the body. This function is performed by enzymes, and enzymes are influenced by minerals—minerals that sugar is working to unbalance.

Enzymes

Most enzymes are mineral-dependent. Minerals work along with enzymes not only to digest food but also to bring about certain necessary biochemical functions in the body.

Chymotrypsin, for example, is a zinc-dependent enzyme needed to fine-tune carbohydrate metabolism, but it's also used to counteract inflammation and bring down swelling.

Every food we eat needs a variety of enzymes to digest and metabolize the food before it can be used by our cells. None of these enzymes will work without the proper minerals to help them out. If the usable minerals in the body decrease, as in the presence of sugar, there will not be enough of them for proper enzyme functions. Therefore, when we ingest sugar, it is difficult for the body to digest anything else that is in the small intestine because of the lack of functioning enzymes. This inability to digest a particular food, over time, results in an allergy to that food. How this occurs is described in the next chapter.

3 | All About Allergies

The word *allergy* carries with it a connotation of sneezes, weepy eyes, and a runny nose. Allergies can be more than that—or something completely different. Allergies are caused by food that is not properly digested. Nutrients cannot be made available to the body, and the lack of nutrients compromises the body's ability to function optimally.

When these undigested food particles enter the bloodstream—due to unbalanced mineral relationships which keep enzymes from functioning properly—they can go to any part of the body and play havoc. If the particles go to the head, the results can be headaches, fatigue, or dizziness; in other parts of the body they cause joint pains, swelling in ankles, legs, or hands, and many other symptoms.

Not coincidentally, the foods most people tend to be allergic to—milk, corn, wheat, and chocolate—are those foods most commonly eaten with sugar. Sugar is added to milk to make ice cream; wheat is blended with sugar in a tempting variety of cookies and cakes; corn in the form of corn sweetener is used to sweeten most processed foods; and chocolate is impossible to eat without some sugar added. It is primarily because we eat these foods so often in large quantities, and so often with sugar, that we are more than likely to become allergic to them.

Another food that commonly causes allergies is eggs, and I am convinced that this is because eggs are eaten with orange juice. A ten-ounce glass of orange juice contains approximately six to eight large whole oranges, the equivalent in simple sugars of nine teaspoons of sugar or a twelve-ounce can of Coke. Many people eat eggs and orange juice day after day, year after year. The simple sugar from the orange juice exhausts the enzymes needed for the eggs, and the eggs then become difficult to digest. Thus, the body develops an allergy to eggs.

It may be hard to believe that orange juice, with all that vitamin C, could do anything bad to the body. In order to prove this theory, I conducted some experiments to see what would happen to the calcium/phosphorus ratio over a four-hour period after orange juice had been ingested. I gave ten ounces of orange juice to two healthy people and found that the orange juice changed the calcium/phosphorus ratio just as plain table sugar did. There seems to be enough simple sugar in ten ounces of orange juice to change the mineral relationships, making it just as harmful as cookies and coffee cake.

If you must have your orange juice for breakfast, drink it when you wake up in the morning. Then get dressed before eating the rest of your breakfast. This will give the juice time to get through your stomach; when the eggs get there, the hydrochloric acid and pepsin in the stomach will be able to digest the protein without the interference of the fruit sugar from the orange juice. You might even try diluting the juice with water, so that you have half juice and half water. Better still, limit the amount of orange juice, apple juice, or other sweet fruit juice that you drink.

Eat the whole fruit instead, and eat it between meals. When you eat the whole fruit, the process of digestion is slowed due to the fiber in the orange. The sugar in the orange doesn't get into the bloodstream quickly; because the process takes longer, it is slowly secreted into the blood. In addition, the fiber works to keep the intestinal track clean and helps with the problem of constipation.

Over thirty years ago, Dr. Theron Randolph, a researcher, learned that people who were allergic to corn reacted more acutely to cooked cornmeal when corn sugar was added than if the cornmeal was eaten alone. The conclusion drawn was that these people were more allergic to sugar than they were to corn. What the researcher didn't realize was that if the corn sugar had been added to any other food the subjects were allergic to, they would have reacted more adversely to the food with the corn syrup in it than without it. Sugar, and this includes corn sugar, depletes enzymes. When there is a deficiency of enzymes, it is possible to become allergic to any undigested food that is sitting in the stomach.

Once a person's body chemistry is unbalanced, any number of life experiences can trigger an allergic response. In fact, our susceptibility to allergies begins at birth. If a mother has nutritional and enzymatic deficiencies, and therefore an unbalanced body chemistry, the body chemistry of her infant may also be unbalanced.

Dr. George Ulett tested the umbilical cord blood of new babies before any food entered the gastrointestinal tract. By cytotoxic testing he found a sensitivity to food to which one or both of the parents were allergic. These sensitivities set the stage for a reaction later on in life. Dr. Ulett felt that in some instances only the allergic tendency was inherited; allergies to specific foods were acquired through exposure. Any food was a potential allergen.

When I was a baby, I threw up my milk every morning. This worried my mother, so she asked my doctor for advice. The doctor told her to let me sleep in the vomit—that this would cure me. It did cure me of vomiting, but it did not cure my body's violent reaction to milk. I was allergic to the milk, but I didn't like sleeping in the vomit, so I adapted.

Or seemingly so. Apparently I didn't adapt very well,

since I had a calcium deposit removed from my chest when I was in college. Milk has a large amount of calcium, and that deposit had been growing since I was a baby. The moral of the story is that I should have listened to my body. The stuffy nose and runny eyes that plagued me as I was growing up were signals of undigested protein, of a reaction of the body to a food that was not being digested. The body constantly tells us things we are unwilling to hear.

If a baby is born with an unbalanced body chemistry, future years may bring on many problems. Dr. Joel Wallach reported a case in which a child developed a rash twelve hours after the nursing mother ate strawberry pie. When the mother stopped eating the pie, the rash went away. When the mother went back to the pie, the infant's rash came back. In Sweden colic in babies was found to occur when the infants' mothers drank milk. It was confirmed immuno-logically that their breast milk contained cow's milk antigen. In Japan the feeding of egg to a nursing mother coincided with the development of eczema in the mother's child.

When a baby is born prematurely, with an undeveloped enzyme system or a deficient enzyme system due to an unbalanced body chemistry, that baby will have more diffi-culty digesting foods. The best way to help a child have a healthy enzyme system and immune system is to breast-feed him or her for the first six months. This is especially important for an allergic baby or one that comes from an allergic family.

Another way we become allergic to a particular food is to eat too much of it at one time. Our enzyme system was not made to handle mounds of mashed potatoes or three glasses of milk at one sitting. When we overeat a food, we use up the specific enzymes for that food. It does not digest as well, and that can cause an allergic reaction. Even a healthful plate of vegetables can be troublesome if you eat more vegetables than you have enzymes. When you feel like binging, it would be wise to go to the best buffet you can find and eat tiny portions of many different foods.

Improperly prepared foods can also cause allergic reactions. Foods such as heated milk and chilled drinks, overcooked foods, fresh or cooked foods that have been stored too long, are all more difficult for the body to digest. A high-protein diet will increase the ammonia levels in the body, and high ammonia levels lead to a toxic state in which nutrients cannot be easily used by the cells.

All protein—whether meat, wheat, or vegetable protein—has the same chemical configuration. Over millions of years, we and our evolutionary ancestors developed enzymes that line up with protein molecules in our intestines. Protein has a heat labile point, at which temperature it becomes denatured and changes its chemical configuration. Because our enzymes are not designed to digest the different configuration, we have trouble digesting protein that has been overcooked. Noxious chemicals cross the intestinal membrane and get into the bloodstream, where the immune system is forced to deal with them. This results in an allergic reaction.

Packaged and processed foods are also hard on the digestive system because they are made for a long shelf life. The longer a food sits before eating, the more depleted the nutrients become. Digestion is hindered by the absence of these nutrients. Unfortunately, processed foods replace the food value with substances the body cannot digest as well.

Some people find that their health, and their ability to digest food without allergic reaction, is never the same after a viral, bacterial, and/or parasitic infection. These infections, or the antibodies needed to combat the infections, seem to compromise the immune system. In many cases these people find themselves allergic to food for the first time. Often they become universal reactors, continually reacting to many items in their environment.

A healthy body is like an orchestra. Just as the string section balances the wind section and so on to make the music sound harmonious, so it is with a healthy body. The thyroid secretes thyroxin, the adrenals secrete adrenaline, and all of the glands secrete small amounts of hormones into the bloodstream so that a balance or harmony is obtained. When heredity, environmental factors, or illness upsets this balance, immune suppression occurs. The use of sugar, day in and day out, over a period of years—and eventually through several generations—can cause a certain degree of atrophy or abnormal functioning of the overworked glands. The more abnormal the functioning, the more food sensitivities can be present if we have an upset body chemistry.

Our polluted environment can cause allergies. Studies show that city air may be three or four thousand times more polluted than sea air. Pollution from car exhaust, industrial pollution, or forestry pesticide spraying can exacerbate food allergies. Indoor air pollution at places of employment adds to the likelihood of environmentally triggered disease. One office was analyzed and found to have four hundred times greater concentrations of chemicals in the air as compared with the outside air. Each threshold limit was below the theoretically safe level for individual exposure to that particular chemical, but the combined and cumulative effects of multiple chemicals had never been evaluated.

The environment of the average home has also been shown to be highly polluted. Fumes from gas heating and cooling appliances, the outgassing of such soft plastics as nylon, polyester, polyurethane, and polyethylene, and routine use of pesticides all contribute to the contamination. Another factor in the total overload is the daily use of chemically contaminated water. A recent analysis of local city water was shown to have 1,000 times more synthetic components than normal.

A friend of mine from England became allergic to most everything in her environment after the gas company changed some gas pipes in her home. For six months she did not know that there were leaks in the pipes which were causing gas to seep into her home. After the leak was found and the food allergens which had accumulated over the past six months were removed from her diet, the woman slowly became well again.

Dr. William J. Rea found that some of his patients developed food allergies after exposure to massive chemicals. Most could eat any food as much and as often as desired before exposure. After exposure it was apparent to many of the patients that the ingestion of foods in general bothered them. After unmasking the foods to which they were allergic and eliminating those foods from their diet, many found that by using meticulous selection of food, they could have a symptom-free meal for the first time in months. In order to remain symptom free, it was clear that these patients had to continue avoiding their symptom producing foods for a period of at least six to twelve months. As their daily chemical exposures decreased, their tolerance increased, and they were able to eat foods previously not tolerated. Furthermore, during visits to areas of significantly lower air pollution, they found that they could tolerate foods to which they were usually susceptible. As you can see, there are no simple reasons why some people get food allergies, nor are there simple cures.

Pollens, gases, hydrocarbons, cats, horses, perfumes, and other substances can upset a person's body chemistry, but only when the body has already been compromised. A massive attack of any one substance can upset anyone's body chemistry, but normal exposure to perfumes, paints, or newsprint will not upset healthy people. When you remove sugar and the offending foods from your diet and stop upsetting your chemistry by stress, your immune system will be rejuvenated and be able to remove those offending inhalant allergies from your body. The inhalant allergies will subside when you stop bombarding your body with foods and stress.

What's Ahead?

More research needs to be done to find out what happens to the body when we eat different foods. Research designed to discover the impact of carbohydrate ingestion usually concerns itself with the rise and fall of blood glucose. Very little examination has been done on what happens to minerals, because very few clinicians today realize that minerals work only in relation to each other.

Much of the money that goes for research on food and disease comes from the food industry or the pharmaceutical industry. The food industry is not interested in supporting research on the effect of sugar on the body, because it relies on sugar for the manufacture of processed foods. The pharmaceutical industry, on the other hand, doesn't participate in non-drug-oriented research. In fact, sugar research would be harmful to the drug industry, because if people stopped eating sugar they wouldn't need so many drugs. Even the limited amount of experimentation in this field has launched a worldwide crusade toward whole foods and the virtual elimination of drugs.

So how exactly does this mineral-enzyme-allergy connection work? When protein digests correctly, it is broken down first into polypeptides and then into amino acids, which are absorbed in the bloodstream. When it does not break down completely, when the enzymes charged with the job are incapable of performing properly due to a mineral deficiency, protein can be absorbed through the intestinal wall and into the bloodstream, reaching tissue in partially digested form. The body's immune system correctly interprets this undigested or "putrefied" protein as foreign matter and goes on the attack, causing an allergic reaction. In the next chapter we'll take a closer look at the complete allergy process, from acute reaction to chronic reaction to degenerative disease. Included along the way are all the typical symptoms of allergy, as well as addiction and the breakdown of the immune system. We'll also see how sugar works directly on the phagocytes, or white blood cells of the immune system, decreasing their ability to absorb bacteria and fight off disease.

4 | The Destruction of the Immune System

In the 1930s a researcher named Dr. Hans Selye began looking at stress and what it does to the body. He observed that when people eat something to which they are allergic, or smell a chemical to which they are reactive, there is an initial alarm reaction—an acute reaction. If the stimulus continues, a stage of adaption follows, lasting from minutes to years. During this stage the symptoms are chronic. Finally, adaption fails and a stage of exhaustion is reached. In this degenerative stage the body enters a disease state and eventually dies.

In his book *Stress Without Distress*, Selye called this progression from acute to chronic to degenerative reaction the Biological Stress Syndrome. This concept is only now being understood and acknowledged by the medical community. It has come to be known as the General Adaption Syndrome. There are many kinds of stress that can affect the body: stress from sugar, stress from food not properly digested, stress from a body out of alignment, and psychological stress, among others.

Cigarette smoking is a good example of an environmental stimulus that sends the body into the General Adaption Syndrome. Many people get dizzy, perspire, and sometimes even throw up when they first start smoking. That is the alarm reaction; the body is allergic to the smoke. Then the body adapts. Smoking no longer causes those initial symptoms. In fact, it begins to feel good to smoke. The smoker is becoming addicted.

The body becomes so accustomed to compensating for the allergy that it will go through withdrawal symptoms if the substance is withdrawn. Finally, often after years of abuse and overwork, the mechanisms responsible for adaption break down and become exhausted. The body is no longer able to protect itself from the harmful substance, and a disease state develops. The particular disease depends on the genetic weaknesses of the individual; it could be cancer, heart disease, lung disease, or a variety of other ailments.

The same thing happens with food allergies. In the previous chapter we saw how a food allergy begins. The overuse of sugar and other foods to which we have become allergic causes a mineral imbalance, which in turn causes an enzyme deficiency. When enzymes are incapable of properly digesting food, bits of undigested protein are able to escape into the bloodstream. The immune system properly recognizes these proteins as intruders, and reacts to them just as it would react to a virus.

When the immune system becomes exhausted through overuse, the symptoms of allergy appear. At this point, there can be an acute reaction such as hay fever, joint pain, headache, or fatigue. If the body continues to be exposed, it proceeds through the other stages of the degenerative disease process: chronic reaction and degenerative reaction. Let's take a closer look at each of these three stages and how they relate to Selye's theory of alarm, adaption, and exhaustion.

Stage I: Acute Reaction

As Selye pointed out, the body's first reaction to a foreign substance (and the body treats a food to which it is allergic as a foreign substance) is one of alarm. This is an acute reaction, an immediate response to a foreign stimulus or substance. The immune system goes into action, with possible redness and swelling internally or externally as the result. The reaction is usually finished shortly, and the body returns to homeostasis.

When an offending food—a food which cannot be properly digested, therefore causing undigested food to enter the bloodstream—is introduced into the body for the first time, the body cannot cope with it. This might be the problem with babies who develop diarrhea, diaper rash, vomiting, colic, or other symptoms. A baby's first experience with homogenized milk, for example, might be an alarm reaction resulting in the throwing up of the milk.

My daughter, Laurie, is the perfect example of this. I was able to breast-feed her only for a month. As my milk decreased and I needed to give her a bottle, she started throwing up the milk. Every time I gave her a bottle, it would come right back up. The guilt that I felt because I could not feed her was painful, and I'm sure that distressed her little body in another way.

The doctor told me just to give her another bottle. It didn't seem right to me even at the time, but I did it. The second bottle usually stayed down; she was adapting. Throwing up the milk was an acute reaction which eventually passed, but other symptoms came to take its place.

If a food to which the body is allergic is continually eaten, the body will adapt. The symptoms of acute reaction disappear, but this does not mean that all is well. The reactions have simply grown more complex and chronic.

Stage II: Chronic Reaction

As the body adapts, the immune system continues to defend the body from undigested protein just at it would from bacteria or a virus. Since the white blood cells of the immune system are made of protein—protein which the body is not getting in a usable form—the system cannot function correctly and soon becomes exhausted. The more the immune system is exposed to the offending food, the less able the white cells are to respond correctly to any "invader." The body becomes susceptible to diseases, both infectious and degenerative.

With the weakening of the white cells, the body's reaction to foods to which it is allergic changes from acute—a quick response from the white cells and a quick return to normal—to chronic. Chronic means slow progress and long continuance; it takes longer for the body to return to homeostasis than in an acute reaction. Joint pains, migraine headaches that last for days, edema, and swollen legs and hands are all chronic reactions, and can all be symptoms of food allergies.

Laurie, for example, had colic every afternoon from the time she was six months to ten months old; her little body was protesting again, this time chronically. As an older child, she had all the symptoms of allergy: eczema, runny nose, and sneezing. Finally we eliminated milk and other foods to which she was allergic from her diet, and all the symptoms disappeared.

Unfortunately, chronic symptoms of food allergy are more usually treated by the medical community with pain medication, tranquilizers, antidepressants, stimulants, anticonvulsants, diuretics, muscle relaxants, nutrients, and even surgical removal of symptom-producing tissue. The best cure, as we found with Laurie, is withdrawal from the offending foods. Nevertheless, each time a person eats these foods, he or she suppresses the immune system and eventually exhausts it.

Babies who are allergic to milk but are continually fed milk over a period of time will learn to keep the milk down. Their resistance to milk becomes diminished, and the original alarm reaction virtually disappears. This stage of adaption is relatively free of symptoms. It can also become a stage of addiction. If these babies don't get milk on a daily basis, they can go through withdrawal symptoms.

In our society we tend to eat a few foods over and over again. Our diet is not varied. Our crops are not rotated. Because of refrigerators and freezers, we can eat the same foods all year. "Fast foods" all contain the same basic elements: wheat, eggs, milk, caffeine, corn, yeast, and, worst of all, sugar. After overeating these foods on a daily basis, a person can become allergy-addicted to some. Most of us don't realize we're addicted; we just know that we feel better when we eat certain foods. We time our meals so as to avoid withdrawal symptoms that come from not eating those foods, whether knowingly or unknowingly. Of course, as we have seen, each time we eat a food to which we've become allergic, we suppress our immune system and eventually exhaust it.

In the adaptive stage of food allergy, a person can have withdrawal symptoms from three hours to three days after exposure to the offensive substance if he or she is not exposed to it again. The body takes a long time to return to normal from its chronic reaction. The only way to avoid the discomfort of that withdrawal is to expose the body to that substance again, to drink that cup of coffee or can of pop, to keep the body in continual reaction. This applies not only to food allergies but to sugar, alcohol, cigarettes, caffeine, and other abusive substances as well.

Many phobias, anxieties, and obsessions develop out of the withdrawal phase of addiction during the adaptive stage. Brain allergies or inflammation in specific areas of the central nervous system can cause emotional reactions from minor to psychotic proportions. An addicted person can become angry, depressed, hyperactive, or withdrawn. When I was in this state, I used to get nervous, impatient, and was apt to fly off the handle at the slightest provocation.

During withdrawal from allergic reactions to foods, chemicals or inhalants, acidosis can occur. Acidosis is that state of imbalance when the body is more acid than alkaline. The body's enzyme functions are dependent not only on minerals but also on a narrow pH range (acid-alkali balance). Therefore, acidosis reduces the enzyme function, which results in still more undigested protein and more allergic reaction. In the acid state the undigested protein (also called peptides and endorphins) might actually initiate addiction because of druglike effects. Some people might recognize this as a feeling of mellowness, others as fatigue or sleepiness. Foods can definitely change how you function, how you think, and how you feel.

The more addicted a person becomes to the food, the more of that food he or she eats, and the more the body is forced to adapt. This leads to an exhaustion of the enzyme system and the immune system, causing the body to move from chronic reaction and adaption to degenerative reaction and disease.

Stage III: Degenerative Reaction

Degenerative disease means a worsening of physical or mental qualities; in the case of such degenerative diseases as cancer, arthritis, and heart disease, the cells and tissues change. The functions of some cells and tissues may be stopped altogether, and the body has a hard time returning to and maintaining homeostasis. Eventually the entire biochemical balance needed for health is destroyed, and continued imbalance is the cause of disease.

Our genetic blueprint decides which disease we will get according to our inherited weakness. My weakness was my chest. First I had pneumonia, a disease of the chest. Then a calcium tumor was removed from my lungs. After a few more bouts with pneumonia, I ended up with chronic bronchitis. I feel very fortunate that I was able to change my life-style and not only stop the degenerative disease process in my lungs but also turn the process around. I was able to eliminate all the phlegm from my chest, and my body healed itself.

The consequences of continuing abuse during the degenerative stage are grave. Let's consider, for example, an individual who is allergic to milk. The body may have adapted to milk, but eventually this ability to adapt will become exhausted. This final exhaustion could be due to an overload in the body of stressors—possibly the person ate too many milk products at one time and overdosed, or drank milk during hay fever season and the two stressors were too much for the body. Milk had been suppressing the body's immune system for a long time, and the individual may have been exposed to excessive heat or cold, fatigue, an infection, or emotional stress.

At this time, the signs that initially appeared upon

contact with the food, or possibly different signs, will reappear. They might take the form of joint pains, bloating, gas, or headaches. If this person does not stop drinking milk or eating milk products, or continues other dietary indiscretions and abusive life-styles, the symptoms will become irreversible. Depending on the affected organs, determined by his or her genetic blueprint, this could result in death. You may never have heard of anyone dying of a milk allergy, but the allergy has so worn down the immune system that the body was susceptible to any disease that came along.

The degenerative disease process now begins because of lack of protein, acidosis, insufficient enzymes, exhaustion of the immune system, and cytotoxic reaction.

This process of allergy, adaption, addiction, and exhaustion is true for any life-style abuse. If you don't stop doing the things that make your body sick, all the medicine, vitamins, and other nutritional supplements in the world won't help make you well.

Some Other Studies

Two different research projects have been done at Loma Linda University to study the effect of sugar on the phagocytic index. The phagocytes are those white blood cells of the immune system that eat up foreign invaders and debris; they're the Pac-Men of the body. The more bacteria eaten by each phagocyte, the stronger the immune system becomes and the less chance of the body becoming diseased. The phagocytic index is the average number of invaders engulfed by a phagocyte.

One of the Loma Linda studies, conducted in 1973, examined what happened to this index when a subject ingested sugar (sucrose), glucose, fructose, honey, orange juice, and starch. Except for the starch, all the substances were simple sugars. The starch was also the only substance which caused a rise in the phagocytic index—the phagocytes actually ate up more bacteria after starch was ingested. The index was highest approximately one half hour after the volunteers ate the starch. The sugars, on the other hand, caused the phagocytic index to decrease greatly. The index was lowest two hours after ingestion. In other words, the sugar had a directly harmful effect on the amount of bacteria removed by the immune system. Figure 4-1 compares the reaction of phagocytes to starch and sugar.

FIGURE 4-1

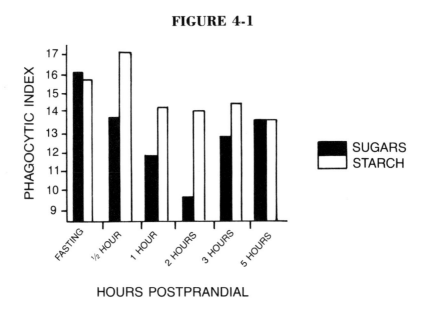

HOURS POSTPRANDIAL

Next, these researchers investigated the effect of fasting on the phagocytic index. They had subjects fast for sixty hours, and the phagocytic capacity to engulf foreign invaders rose from 11 per phagocyte to 16. Fasting seems to strengthen the immune system, as shown in Figure 4-2. The researchers did not check for food allergens, but if they had, and removed those from the diets of these volunteers, possibly the phagocytic index before fasting would have been as high as after fasting.

FIGURE 4-2

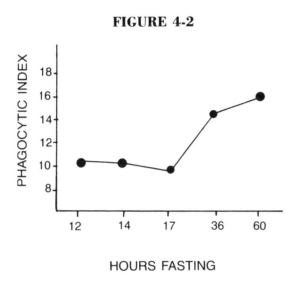

HOURS FASTING

This corresponds to the findings of an earlier Loma Linda study, conducted in 1964, which proved that the higher the fasting blood glucose in diabetics, the lower the phagocytic index. Diabetes is an inability of the body to metabolize sugar properly, with the result that excess sugar appears in the blood and the urine. Even when fasting, diabetics have higher blood glucose than nondiabetics, and this glucose in the blood works to suppress the immune system. As a result, statistics show that diabetics are more susceptible to diseases than nondiabetics; they are more likely to have heart and blood disease, kidney and liver dysfunction, and eye problems, as well as infectious diseases.

These researchers also studied the actions of individual

phagocytes under a microscope to observe the specific changes that occurred in the presence of sugar. Where the glucose level was normal, the phagocytic cells were very active. Pseudopods (little arms that reach out from the cell) extended in all directions in search of foreign objects. The higher the amount of sugar in the blood, however, the less active the cells became. An increasing amount of fat was observed in the cell, resulting in slower, sluggish action of the phagocytes toward foreign objects.

Both of these studies addressed themselves to the problems of sugar in the diet. In this book I focus specifically on the effect of sugar on mineral relationships; the Loma Linda researchers looked at sugar's effect on the immune system. Our conclusions are the same. Through the combined effects of mineral imbalance, allergic reaction, and phagocytic suppression, sugar destroys the immune system and slowly but surely leads to degenerative disease.

In the next chapter we'll take a closer look at these degenerative diseases.

5 | The Consequences

The current life expectancy in the United States is over seventy-four years, up from forty-nine years at the turn of the century. This increase seems miraculous, but those extra years have been almost wholly gained in the early years of life. Improved hospital conditions have reduced the number of deaths at birth, while polio, chicken pox, and other childhood diseases have been brought under control. When these figures are included, the "average" person appears to live longer. The life expectancy of the average fifty-year old male today is only two years longer than it was a hundred years ago. That is, once a male has attained the age of fifty, all the achievements of modern medicine extend his life only eighteen months over his counterpart of a century ago. In terms of diseases of older people—arthritis, cancer, heart disease, and others—not much headway has been made.

In the previous chapters we've seen how sugar sets about unbalancing the body's mineral relationships and immune system. This damage, done by sugar, manifests itself in many degenerative diseases and harmful conditions.

Those which are discussed briefly in this chapter are: hypoglycemia, hyperglycemia (diabetes), constipation, gas, asthma, headaches, psoriasis, cancer, arthritis, candida overgrowth, obesity, heart disease, osteoporosis, tooth decay, multiple sclerosis, inflammatory bowel disease, canker sores, gallstones, and cystic fibrosis.

It should be noted that these conditions in their less serious stages can degrade the quality of one's life, producing those feelings of, "I don't really fell well, but I'm not really sick." To whatever extent these conditions affect you, that extent can be greatly decreased by a healthy diet and life-style.

Hypoglycemia

The first endocrine organ to come into contact with ingested foods or chemicals is the pancreas. A hormone secreted by the pancreas is responsible for controlling the amount of sugar in the bloodstream. Malfunctioning of the pancreas can cause either excessively low or abnormally high levels of sugar in the blood. Therefore, it is not surprising that of all the endocrine glands, the pancreas is the most susceptible to damage by excess sugar. When we ingest sugar, our blood sugar level goes up. Clusters of endocrine cells in the pancreas, called the islets of Langerhans, detect this excess sugar in the blood and secrete a hormone, insulin, which brings the blood sugar level back down to normal. When sugar is eaten and overeaten obsessively for a number of years, the pancreas can become overstimulated and secrete too much insulin. Excess insulin can make the blood sugar drop below normal, and hypoglycemia (low blood sugar) may develop.

The islets of Langerhans secrete another hormone called

glucagon, which stimulates the release of glycogen, a sugar stored in the liver and tissues. This mechanism can wear out from overuse, and glycogen may not be released. The individual then goes into a hypoglycemic state, and may eat more sugar to keep the sugar level normal, which in turn causes further destruction.

An interesting phenomenon that many physicians have discovered is that abnormally high (hyperglycemia) or abnormally low (hypoglycemia) blood sugar levels can occur in a person who has eaten a food or come in contact with a chemical to which he or she is sensitive. These can include fats, carbohydrates, proteins, inhalants, and tobacco, and are specific to each individual. When the allergy-provoking substance is removed, the blood sugar level returns to normal.

Hypoglycemia is an adaptive stage of this allergic reaction; as the endocrine cells adapt to excess sugar or allergic substances, they begin to secrete too much insulin. Symptoms that might occur during a hypoglycemic state include fatigue (usually a few hours after sugar is ingested), falling asleep after meals, memory failure, rapid heartbeat, anxieties, tremors, hunger pangs, giddiness, headaches, perspiration, and depression.

Although it was a long time ago, I still vividly remember driving home one day after having lunch with a friend, feeling weak and dizzy and perspiring heavily. I didn't think I'd had that much sugar—I'd just had a meringue dessert with a couple of cups of coffee—but what I didn't realize is that when the homeostatic mechanisms of the body aren't working correctly, the caffeine in coffee can drop the blood sugar level as well as sugar. So between the coffee and the meringue, I was in bad shape. These symptoms of hypoglycemia are not very pleasant, yet many people experience them day after day without really dealing with them; they think it's all in their head, or that they just have to live with the problem. In fact, removing all junk food from your diet is a great start toward removing these symptoms. As scary as these symptoms are, what's even more scary is what this life-style does internally to the immune system, the glands, and the organs of the body.

Diabetes

If hypoglycemia is the adaptive stage of an allergic reaction, then hyperglycemia (diabetes) is the exhaustive stage. As with other overstimulated tissues and organs, the overworked pancreas eventually wears out and stops functioning correctly. The islets of Langerhans become exhausted and slow down or stop the secretion of insulin. The body can no longer adapt, as it did in hypoglycemia, and diabetes is the result.

Even if the islets continue to secrete insulin at a normal rate, that insulin may be too weak to do any good. As we saw in Chapter 2, sugar causes a calcium/phosphorus imbalance which renders the body incapable of breaking down proteins into amino acids—the essential building blocks of hormones. Without protein, insulin begins to diminish; the resulting insulin deficiency can also cause hyperglycemia and diabetes.

There are two types of diabetes. The first, juvenile onset or Type 1 diabetes, is characterized by a complete lack of insulin in the islets of Langerhans. "Juvenile onset" doesn't mean that just children can get it; adults, too, can get this type of diabetes. There is a possibility that Type 1 is transmitted by a virus. Ten percent of all diabetics have Type 1 diabetes.

Far more common is Type 2, adult onset diabetes, and it is this type which we will be concentrating on here. In Type 2 diabetes, insulin is in the cells of the islets of Langerhans, but an insufficient amount of insulin is being secreted. The insulin being secreted is not of good quality or the body is unable to use properly the insulin that the pancreas secretes. The mechanism for moving the insulin out of the cells and into the bloodstream has malfunctioned, and the levels of glucose in the blood remain high after a carbohydrate has been ingested. Some Type 2 diabetics have symptoms similar to Type 1—frequent urination, extreme thirst, ravenous hunger, weight loss, extreme fatigue, loss of concentration, memory failure, dizziness, unprovoked anxiety, tremors, cuts that are slow to heal, frequent skin infections, headaches—while others have no symptoms at all.

Research shows that as sugar in the diet increases, there is an increased urinary excretion of chromium. Many diabetics have shown to be deficient in chromium. When this happens, other minerals cannot function as well.

Many doctors today don't seem to feel that there is a correlation between how much sugar one eats and diabetes, but as sugar consumption has increased in the United States, so has diabetes proportionally. During World War II, when sugar consumption dropped, the outbreak of diabetes dropped sharply also.

Dr. John Potts tested diabetics for reactive foods and found that two thirds of the Type 2 diabetics did not need artificial insulin after they had withdrawn from foods to which they were allergic. Those who still required insulin needed only one third as much, once they removed reactive foods from their diets.

In another experiment a group of volunteers increased their sugar consumption for six weeks so that it would be 40 percent of their diet (not, unfortunately, unlike the diet of many teenagers). Testing of blood sugar levels and insulin levels before and after the six weeks showed higher levels of glucose and insulin, both while fasting and after sugar ingestion, in the blood of the volunteers. Clearly, then, the mechanism that controls blood glucose becomes faulty when there are high levels of sugar in the diet.

The overeating of concentrated refined foods, including sugar and white flour, puts added strain on the pancreas and the production of insulin. Sugar goes into the bloodstream quickly. The more refined foods are ingested, the more danger to the pancreas. It may take as long as twenty years for diabetes to develop. Maintaining normal weight, exercising, and eating foods to which a person is not reactive and of course eating no refined sugar seem to be four simple steps in controlling Type 2 diabetes.

Constipation

Not only does sugar put a strain on the pancreas, but it has ramifications for other endocrine glands as well. When we continually overeat sugar and our blood sugar rises, the insulin level in our blood also has to rise. The thyroid gland must secrete a hormone, thyroxin, into the bloodstream to open the receptor cells and let the insulin into the cells. Eventually the thyroid itself becomes exhausted, and since the thyroid regulates metabolic functions, everything in the body slows down. Nutrient-rich blood moves through the body more slowly. Blood pressure is lowered, making it all the more difficult for nutrients to move through the body. The feces also move through the body too slowly, and this can cause constipation.

Eating sugar over and over can lead to constipation in other ways. We've seen how sugar inhibits enzymes; when enzymes aren't working, undigested food putrifies in the small intestine. Inflammation sets in to protect the lining of the small intestine and colon from the undigested proteins. This inflammation makes the passage smaller and more difficult for the feces to move through, and the mucus that forms makes it nearly impossible for nutrients to reach the bloodstream.

If sugar and white flour are a large part of your diet, you're lacking not only nutrients but also fiber and bulk. Lack of fiber has been implicated in colon cancer because the feces stay in the colon too long, and the bacteria that are supposed to be quickly eliminated from the body are not. They seep back into the walls of the colon and become toxic to the body. When there is no fiber to make bulk, the feces become hard and do not move along quickly through the colon. Hard feces can stick to the lining of the colon and cause diverticulitis, colitis, and other diseases.

If you are suffering from constipation, you might consider making the following changes in your diet:

1. Eliminate all refined foods.

2. Eat lots of raw foods and vegetables.

3. Exercise (preferably aerobics) at least twenty minutes a day, five days a week.

4. Drink more water (six to eight glasses a day).

5. Do not neglect the calls of nature. You might find that half an hour later nature is no longer calling.

6. Eat only a small amount of animal protein at one meal and chew thoroughly. There will be less opportunity for protein to putrify in the colon.

7. Watch out for iron supplements. If you need to take them and are having constipation problems, try a different form of iron to find out if your constipation lessens.

8. Avoid all commercial laxatives. Use herbal laxatives sold in health food stores with senna pods or senna leaf tea, flax, psyllium seed, or cascara sagrada.

9. Avoid coffee, tea, and alcohol. They have been found to be constipating for many people.

10. Make sure you get two tablespoons of vegetable oil a day (preferably cold-pressed).

11. Eat a high-fiber diet. There are three types of fiber: bran, pectin, and guar. Make sure your diet has the bran from whole grains, the pectin from fruits, and guar from beans. Also include root vegetables and leafy green ones.

There are many cleansing programs recommended by various companies that manufacture supplements. These consist of bulking agents, herbs, vitamins and minerals, all of which help to pull putrefied materials from the colon; creams to rub on the colon area to stimulate the colon; and enzymes to take at meals to keep more putrefied foods from collecting in the colon.

Many programs are good. Keep two things in mind when deciding which program to use. The first is that most programs recommend fruit juice, but many people are sugar-sensitive. The program could do more harm than good. Use vegetable juices instead or just spring water.

The second thing to remember is that you might be allergic to one of the items in the program. Take each supplement and test it individually to find out if your body reacts to it. Take one in the morning on an empty stomach. Take your pulse before and ten minutes after to see if it goes up ten beats per minute; this indicates sensitivity. Watch out for symptoms during the first hour. You can use the calcium-urine test if you have a kit (see Chapter 8) to test for allergies.

Don't forget that if you resume the consumption of refined foods, your colon can again become clogged. Concentrate on changing your dietary habits to keep your body in harmony and functioning optimally.

Stomach or Intestinal Gas

Gas forms whenever food does not digest properly. It is therefore another clear signal of an unbalanced body chemistry. Stomach gas is usually caused by too much or too little hydrochloric acid in the stomach. If gas occurs immediately after swallowing the food, this indicates a high level of hydrochloric acid. If gas forms from one to several hours later, or is present the morning after eating the food, a deficiency in hydrochloric acid is indicated. Intestinal gas can be due to disturbed liver and pancreatic functions as well as a low hydrochloric acid level. A very active liver or an underactive pancreas makes for an acid stool, and whenever stools are too alkaline or too acidic, gas is produced.

If gas is a problem for you, following the suggestions on this list can help you correct it.

1. Eat small amounts of protein at each meal, about two ounces.

2. Eat all your protein at the beginning of the meal, followed by vegetables and then carbohydrates.

3. Eat your meals slowly.

4. Eliminate foods—such as beans (especially baked and lima), onions, radishes, turnips, yams, parsnips, lettuce hearts, and sugar—which are known to cause gas in some people.

5. Chew each bite of food at least twenty times.

6. Don't drink water during meals—you'll dilute your hydrochloric acid.

7. Eat fruit between meals only.

8. Use the calcium-urine test (Chapter 8) or other means to check for foods to which you are reactive, as these can cause gas. Eliminate these foods from your diet.

Arthritis

Arthritis is a painful inflammatory disease found in many people. Rheumatoid arthritis is inflammation in the joints; osteoarthritis is inflammation in the bones and cartilage. There is considerable evidence that people who are allergic to certain foods build what are called immune complexes in their blood. These immune complexes are a combination of food to which we are allergic and a protective substance, called an antibody, which our body makes to defend us against what the body considers a foreign invader. As these foreign substances are glued together by the antibodies, an immune complex develops. These complexes, which often collect in the joints, cause tissue damage and inflammation, partly from the release of free radicals, the by-product of the immune complexes. As we know, food allergy does not develop unless a body is out of homeostasis. A body which has been compromised, due to mineral imbalance, is unable to make enzymes to remove the free radicals from the body. Inflammation in the bones and cartilage can be caused by an accumulation of toxic minerals, mostly calcium. This, too, is caused by a body out of balance.

Dr. William Catterall points out in an article in *Arthritis News Today* that, in over 232 cases from four independent investigators, the following observations were made: (1) With few exceptions, when a restricted (or fasting) diet was followed, acute arthritic symptoms disappeared. (2) Symptoms developed when certain foods were individually restored to the diet. (3) Symptoms disappeared again when each one of such foods was withdrawn. (4) Most patients experienced several cycles of symptom production and remission in response to foods. The connection between symptoms and ingestion of offending foods was forcefully and repeatedly demonstrated.

Arthritic patients often have symptoms such as fatigue, weakness, and fever, which are also symptomatic of allergy addiction and withdrawal. Many people with food allergy symptoms get worse during the night or early in the morning, perhaps accounting for arthritic morning stiffness.

Once again we see that if we stop doing to the body what makes it sick, the body will heal itself.

Asthma

The original meaning of asthma was heavy difficulty in breathing, but now the word is taken to mean a particular kind of difficulty arising from spasm of involuntary muscle around the small branches of the air tubes (bronchi) in the lungs.

In the past, asthmatic attacks have been ascribed to three main causes: allergy, infection, and emotional disturbance. Some recent research has shown that food allergy plays a large role in asthma.

A report from Israel indicated that of twenty-two patients with asthma, fifteen improved remarkably within weeks after avoiding all dairy foods. When the fifteen patients were then challenged with dairy products, five had recurrence of severe asthma attacks.

Unfortunately the article didn't say whether the authors tested people for other food allergies. Food allergies are individual to each person. With more information concerning foods to which they reacted, more of the asthmatics would have been helped.

After a study of over a year, researchers from the Netherlands concluded that the involvement of allergic foods with bronchial asthma is more frequent than traditionally assumed. Ninety-eight percent of 110 patients showed distinct decrease of asthmatic complaints with avoidance of allergic foods for six to twelve months.

The detective work for asthmatics called for extensive research because three types of bronchial responses were observed: immediate responses (onset within twenty to forty-five minutes, with resolution within two hours after food challenge), late response (onset within four to six hours, resolving within twenty-four hours), and delayed type (onset within twenty-eight to thirty-two hours, resolving within forty-eight to fifty-six hours after food challenge). An asthmatic might best work with a clinician to help with detective work and support the patient during this trying time.

Headaches

For years, articles have been written on foods in relation to headaches. Caffeine has been implicated because it restricts the blood vessels. Tyramine-containing foods have also been suggested as headache causes. These foods include cheese, organ meats, alcohol, chocolate, yogurt, and smoked and aged meats. Monosodium glutamate (MSG) is a substance which can cause different symptoms in people, including headaches. MSG is found in many Oriental and processed foods.

In one recent study, done at Charing Cross Hospital in London, wheat caused headaches in 78 percent of the people tested, oranges in 65 percent, eggs in 45 percent, tea and coffee in 40 percent, chocolate and milk in 37 percent, beef in 35 percent, and corn, cane sugar, and yeast in 3 percent each. When these eleven common foods were avoided, there was a dramatic fall in the number of headaches per month; 85 percent of the patients became headache-free.

My professional experience has been that any food can cause headaches. Moreover, attacks do not follow the same pattern in each person. Each food must be tested individually by withdrawing the food for four days, reintroducing the food and looking for symptoms, through the cytotoxic test or the urine kit (Chapter 8). When the headache-causing foods are withdrawn from the diet, the person may go through withdrawal symptoms. When the foods have been removed from the body for three or four days, the headache sufferer experiences relief. Attacks do not follow the same pattern in each person. Headache attacks could appear immediately after the offending food or be delayed for as much as twenty-four hours or more.

Psoriasis

Psoriasis is a skin disease which manifests itself in large scaly patches which appear anywhere on the body or all over the body. Usually when psoriasis is present, the liver is not functioning correctly, and therefore a liver-cleansing program is a good place to start. The cleansing program that is used for constipation can also be used for the liver (see pages 46–48). The body chemistry has been compromised and each person needs to find out what he has been doing to upset his body.

Dr. John M. Douglass, from Kaiser Permanente Medical Group in Los Angeles, has used elimination diets to improve the condition of his psoriasis patients. Douglass asked his patients to stop using such acid foods as coffee, tomatoes, sodas, and pineapple. The result was a great improvement in his clients.

When the liver is functioning well and reactive foods have been eliminated from the diet, there are excellent results. This is not a rapid process. The program needs to be followed for many months, but preliminary results can be seen within a few weeks.

Cancer

Statistics show that one out of three people today will get cancer. Cancer is a condition in which normal cells turn abnormal—they turn cancerous. It is clearly important to have some understanding of the process which permits cancer to occur. A theory which relies upon the nutritional ideas described in this book is given below. These ideas can greatly help you and your doctor battle cancer.

In 1920 Dr. Otto Walberg took human cells and removed 35 percent of the oxygen from the cells, and they became cancerous. He then put oxygen back into the cells, and they did not become normal again. His conclusion was that cancer is not reversible. Walberg was apparently right to the extent that the cells will turn cancerous if 35 percent of the oxygenation potential of the cells is taken away. However, he apparently was not right in his conclusion, because it has been shown that cancerous cells do turn back to normal.

One way to turn cells cancerous is continually to upset the body chemistry. In normal body chemistry the cell develops by-products called free radicals. These poisonous by-products include peroxide, hydroxyl group, and superoxide.

We also have enzymes in our body that treat these free radicals and turn them back into useful products. The enzymes are peroxidase, catalase, and superoxide dismutase. As we have learned, enzymes depend on minerals in order to function. For example, peroxidase is a selenium-dependent enzyme.

If you continually unbalance your body chemistry by eating sugar or other abusive foods, burning the candle at both ends by go-go-go, distress, anger, rage, and other life-style abuses, you will increase your metabolic rate and produce more free radicals. You will also inhibit peroxidase, superoxide dismutase, and catalase, and the free radicals will build up in your system. When they build up in the system, they interfere with the oxygenation process. When you interfere with 35 percent of the oxygenation process, your cells will turn cancerous.

There are other factors involved with this process also. If you were born with a genetic blueprint causing your endocrine system to oversecrete estrogen, but you keep yourself healthy, you will be an emotionally sensitive person. If you have a genetic blueprint causing you to oversecrete growth hormone from an overactive anterior pituitary, but you are healthy, you will be a big, sensitive person.

A good example of this appears to be Rosie Grier. He is a big man with an overactive anterior pituitary, and he also secretes a large amount of estrogen. He manifests this genetic blueprint as a sensitive man, a good actor, a person who likes to do needlepoint, and also happens to have been a terrific football player. His sensitivity makes him no less a man, but if he starts upsetting his chemistry, he will start interfering with the oxygenation of cells. Too much estrogen will accumulate around the cells, and the cells will become unhappy and turn cancerous.

When you upset your chemistry often enough, many of your 63 trillion cells can't oxygenate; they cannot metabolize properly. The cells say, "Why should I function properly when you treat me like this?"

Cancer cells have a protective coating around them because they know they are going to be attacked by the immune system. The immune system is already being compromised by the person; that is why the cells turn cancerous in the first place. If a person doesn't change the life-style that made him sick, the sick cells start winning— the cancer cells start taking over the body.

Cancer is a creative act. We work hard for our cancer. John Wayne, our national movie hero, worked hard for his cancer and we all encouraged him: "Go get 'em, John." He was very judgmental, smoked his cigars, and drank his booze. He was a symbol for right and wrong for all of us. He had too much estrogen; he was a strong man; he had too much growth hormone; he was a big man. He blew his chemistry long enough to realize the disease expression of his genetic blueprint. While he was younger and healthier, he experienced the health of his genetic blueprint. Had he known this context of thinking, the results might have been much different.

John Wayne's genes didn't cause his disease—upsetting his body chemistry caused his disease. No one's genetic blueprint causes diseases. It is the genetic blueprint that determines what disease will develop out of unbalanced body chemistry. This concept forces us to recognize that we are responsible for our disease. It puts the monkey on our back.

Osteoporosis

As we have seen, sugar causes the phosphorus level in the blood to drop while raising the calcium level. Since these two minerals work in relation to each other, only that calcium which is in the proper ratio to phosphorus is available to the body. Nevertheless, many doctors persist in treating osteoporosis as a simple calcium deficiency, and treat it with calcium supplements. This will work for some people if there is enough phosphorus in the blood to balance the extra calcium. If there is more calcium than can work in ratio with the phosphorus, the supplemental calcium will not help at all. Instead, the supplemental calcium will become toxic.

Stomach acid is another crucial factor in calcium absorption and, ultimately, in bone health. Calcium is absorbed in the upper part of the small intestine, and acid is essential for this process. That's why the frequent use of antacid wreaks havoc on bones. Stomach acid production decreases as we grow older and may be one of the reasons why the efficiency of calcium absorption declines with age. Children absorb 75 percent of the calcium they take in; adults absorb only 30 to 50 percent.

One look at the average American diet should be enough to see that most calcium deficiency is not due to a lack of calcium in the diet. We are getting more calcium than ever before by eating more calcium-rich milk products— milk shakes, pizzas, crepes, cheeseburgers, fruit yogurts, ice cream cones, cheesecakes, and the like. Although there is indeed plenty of calcium in these products, and many other vitamins and minerals also, the nutrients are not so readily available to the body because of the sugar which accompanies them.

When you eat ice cream, for example, you are certainly getting a healthy dose of calcium. However, the sugar in the ice cream lowers the phosphorus in the blood, and the calcium can become toxic rather than useful. Even if the ice cream contained 400 milligrams of calcium, that calcium would metabolize incorrectly and become toxic, or else be secreted in the urine. In addition, refined sugar eaten with milk can bring about a deficiency in the enzyme lactase, which in turn causes an allergy to milk, making the body unable to digest and absorb the milk and you become allergic to milk and other foods. Every time you drink that milk or eat that food to which you are sensitive, you change your calcium/phosphorus ratio. Little calcium is assimilated from the milk products, and the blood turns to the bones for the calcium it needs.

Other substances in the diet can affect the body's ability to absorb calcium. Caffeine, for example—just three cups of caffeinated coffee can make you excrete forty-five milligrams of calcium. The same thing happens with caffeinated tea and soft drinks. Even if the soft drink is sugar-free and caffeine-free, it still contains phosphoric acid, which will also disrupt the calcium/phosphorus ratio.

There seems to be a correlation between cigarette smoking and osteoporosis—several studies have shown that at least three quarters of the women who develop osteoporosis are or were smokers, and most of them smoke or smoked a pack or more a day. Certain medications can also interfere with calcium availability. They include the blood-thinner heparin, diuretics, aluminum-containing antacids, convulsant medications, large doses of thyroid hormone, and corticosteroids used over a long time.

Excess sodium causes loss of calcium in the urine. When calcium is excreted in urine, blood levels of calcium drop. This causes the parathyroid hormone to be released, which breaks down bone in an effort to restore the level of calcium to the blood.

One harmful substance that we don't think of in terms of food consumption is aluminum, which can enter the body through several sources: aluminum in water softeners; alum in cheeses and pickles; aluminum cookware, containers, and foil (watch out for the foil-covered potatoes served in restaurants; don't put your fork through the aluminum); and aluminum in deodorants and toothpastes. This substance, which is now being linked to Alzheimer's disease, can also decrease calcium absorption.

Anything that inhibits the body's ability to absorb calcium contributes to the likelihood of osteoporosis. Sugar is the main dietary culprit—sugar eaten as a child, sugar eaten as a teenager, and sugar eaten in adulthood. It may take decades for the disease to manifest itself in the tissues and bones, and the process starts slowly, usually with neckaches and/or back pains. Chronic pain, the result of a phosphorus deficiency, soon sets in. A chiropractor is needed to put the body back in alignment over and over again. Calcium is drained from the bones, and every time calcium is pulled across the cell membrane—such as when sugar is ingested—protein may be pulled as well. A lack of usable protein indicates that the tissues and bones are being compromised, and the disease progresses.

Then the victim falls down or slips on a stair and breaks a hip. The slightest provocation causes injury. A disc rarefies and gets spongy, and a surgeon must remove it. The simple task of reaching over to tie a shoe causes a pinched nerve, and inflammation sets in. Since the body is unable to heal itself, that inflammation becomes a disease. Doctors are forced to use cortisone to stop the inflammation, and a vicious circle begins.

All these results are reversible. Stop upsetting mineral relationships, and the body will heal itself. I have an easy way of finding out whether my phosphorus is low and if I'm deficient in functioning calcium. When I wake up in the middle of the night or in the morning, I point my toes. If my legs or feet start to cramp, I know I'm low in calcium. This doesn't happen to all people who are deficient in calcium, but it certainly happens to me. I then think about the things I did and the foods I ate the day before, and try to understand how I upset my mineral relationships.

Symptoms vary from person to person. Because calcium is necessary to many heart functions, some people get heart palpitations when their calcium level drops. Other symptoms of calcium deficiency include insomnia, nervousness, arm and leg numbness, rheumatism, arthritis, menstrual cramps, premenstrual cramps, menopausal problems, nervousness, finger tremors, backaches, bone pain, and plaque on the teeth.

Some forms of calcium are more easily digested than others. The calcium supplements that are the most easily absorbable in the body are calcium chelate, calcium orotate, and calcium ascorbate. Also, calcium is not readily taken in by the cell unless accompanied by magnesium. This is because the cell prefers to maintain a ratio of two parts of magnesium to every three parts of calcium. Thus, to offer to the cell membrane a straight calcium compound without magnesium is to ask it to alter its normal ratios, which it is not inclined to do. Therefore, the cell tends to reject the unescorted calcium, which goes out in the urine or stool. Today the preferred ratio of calcium to magnesium in a supplement is one to one.

Periodontal disease (pyorrhea) and gum disorders are forms of osteoporosis of the mouth. As a nutritional consultant, I see many people with osteoporosis or periodontal disease, and in each case excess calcium is being secreted in the urine. There is a simple test you can perform at home to see if you are doing the same (see Chapter 8). To combat osteoporosis in the mouth, or anywhere else, it is essential to stop consuming those items which cause calcium to become deficient and/or toxic, such as ice cream, fruit yogurt, tea, coffee, cigarettes, and products containing aluminum. A reduction in the amount of protein eaten at one meal is also wise; people who have followed a vegetarian diet for twenty years or more, both men and women, show less bone loss than those who eat meat. If you are allergic to milk products, you must stop consuming those as well.

It is still possible to get plenty of calcium in your diet even if you must restrict your intake of milk and milk products. Other foods that are heavy in calcium include sardines, canned salmon, dark green leafy vegetables (collards, kale, turnip greens, mustard greens, and broccoli), Brazil nuts, tofu and all soy products, sunflower seeds, and hulled sesame seeds. There is as much calcium in a glass of carrot juice as in a glass of milk, and it is much more absorbable for many people. Remember—when your minerals are in good relationship and functioning efficiently, your body can absorb all the nutrients in the food you eat. Many foods have small amounts of calcium, and your body will be able to absorb all of it. There are other ways to increase the calcium in your body, always providing that your phosphorus level is high enough to accommodate the additional calcium.

Exercise is the only way short of potent medication to significantly increase bone mass after you have stopped growing. As with muscles, stress (not distress) on the bones strengthens them. Activities that stress the long bones in the body, such as rope jumping, tennis, jogging, walking, cycling, basketball, and dancing are all effective in preventing osteoporosis. One study showed that women who exercised for one hour a day, three days a week for one year, actually gained body calcium, whereas a comparison group of sedentary women lost calcium. If in addition you are getting your exercise outside in the sun, you will get a good dose of vitamin D, which is needed for the absorption of calcium in the body.

There is some controversy today as to whether estrogen is an advantage or disadvantage for menopausal women. Women who are treated with estrogen supplements are less likely to lose significant amounts of bone, but only if the treatment continues for ten to fifteen years. This introduces different risks, as it may promote the growth of cancer in the uterus, breast, and other organs. To reduce the probability of cancer, estrogen therapy should be given in conjunction with progesterone, mimicking the natural premenopausal hormone cycle. Still, many experts say certain women should not take postmenopausal hormone therapy, among them women who have had cancers of the breast or reproductive organs, or who have a family history of these cancers.

The safest way, then, to stop bone loss and maintain adequate calcium in the body is to keep the minerals in balance through proper nutrition and elimination of harmful foods. I have seen postmenopausal women go from secreting calcium twenty-four hours a day to normal in a few weeks (see the program outlined in Chapter 8). It's the same story— balance the minerals in the body and the body will heal itself.

Heart Disease

Heart and blood vessel disease affects one out of every two persons in the United States. There is much new research which indicates a link between sugar and heart disease. The average daily sugar intake of patients with coronary and peripheral vascular diseases is higher (113 to 128 grams) than that of healthy subjects in a control group (58 grams). As Dr. John Yudkin points out: "A person...who is taking more than 120 grams of sugar a day [4 ounces or 8 tablespoons; a Coke has 3 tablespoons] is perhaps five or more times as likely to develop myocardial infarction [clotting of the coronary artery in the heart] as one taking less than 60 grams."

Much of this is due to sugar's unbalancing of the body's chemistry and mineral relationships. Dr. William Philpott found that people who die of coronary artery disease—arteriosclerosis—have no detectable amount of chromium present in their aortas, while those who die accidentally and manifest no coronary artery disease do have chromium present in their aortas. This is directly attributable to sugar; our bodies need chromium to digest sugar. Since sugar contains no chromium, it must be leached from the body.

In a study of eleven men, when 10 percent of the calories that they ate as fat were substituted for glucose, there was a statistically significant increase of blood triglycerides and a decrease in high-density lipoproteins. High-density lipoproteins protect us from heart disease.

Research presented on April 29, 1985, in Miami, at the American Chemical Society's 189th national meeting, suggests that it is the quality of cholesterol in the diet, not the quantity, that contributes most to the risk of developing coronary heart disease and atherosclerosis (hardening of the arteries). In the past, conventional thought has implicated a diet rich in fat with human heart disease. The research suggests that those fats might present a serious hazard only if and when they are transformed through oxidation.

Fred A. Kummerow, a food chemist for the University of Illinois, states that all lipids are unstable and will eventually oxidize. He states that cooking will just speed the process. Kummerow showed that oxidized lipids are toxic to arterial cells.

In one in-vitro test, both partially oxidized cholesterol and partially oxidized vitamin D (also a lipid) decreased the cells' ability to keep out calcium. The researchers claim that not only will too much calcium kill cells, but calcium deposits also characterize advanced atherosclerotic lesions. Dr. Hans Selye found that he could stress rats and give them heart disease, and then, by giving them extra magnesium and potassium, reduce some of the problem. In my practice I have seen the normalization of blood pressure, cholesterol level, and triglyceride level of many people by removing sugar and the foods to which they react from their diets. Your life-style and your diet do have a direct impact on your susceptibility to heart disease, and indeed to all degenerative disease.

We've talked a lot about the calcium/phosphorus ratio and how it is upset by sugar intake. Current medical research has implicated both an excess and a deficiency of calcium in heart disease. This certainly suggests, even to the untrained observer, that calcium should not be considered by itself in bodily processes.

The calcium/magnesium ratio is important too. According to researcher R. J. Doisy, "If calcium and magnesium intakes are high, or the balance between them is optimal, then there is a synergism between them such that both elements are better absorbed. Magnesium, for example, has a protective effect on the atherogenic score in rats only when the diet was high in calcium. Increasing the calcium content of animal diets, coupled with low magnesium intake, is detrimental to these animals. . . . I would like to advance the thesis that it is not only the absolute levels of magnesium that are important; the calcium-magnesium ratio should also be considered. That is, when the ratio is less than two to one, coronary heart disease and diabetes are less prevalent than when the ratio is higher."

Philpott goes on to say that magnesium, calcium, and chromium are a biochemical team which must be present in order for humans to resist the onslaughts of degenerative disease. Copper is also a factor. McKenzie and Kay have demonstrated that individuals with hypertension excrete over two and a half times more copper in their urine than control groups with no hypertension. Many see that there is a correlation between a deficiency in minerals and disease, but few connect this deficiency to undigested food and enzymes. Each one of those little enzymes needs different minerals to function, and when just one is deficient, it upsets the body chemistry and all mineral relationships. Lipids in foods are likely to oxidize in a number of situations, including when cooked meats are stored for some time before eating (even when refrigerated); when prepared foods, such as dehydrated eggs in cake mixes, are processed at extremely high temperature; and when food is cooked in recycled oil that has been heated for a long time, such as potato chips, fried chicken and French fried potatoes, zucchini and onions.

Many of you may have changed from sugar to fructose because of studies showing that fructose is absorbed only 40 percent as quickly as glucose, and causes only a modest rise in blood sugar. Dr. J. Hallfrisch studied cholesterol and triglyceride levels and found that fructose unfortunately caused a general increase in both the total serum cholesterol level and the low-density lipoprotein fraction of cholesterol in most subjects. The triglyceride levels also rose significantly, especially in those persons whose blood sugar levels rise higher than normal when they eat sugar. It was concluded that high levels of dietary fructose can produce undesirable changes in blood lipid levels, which are associated with heart disease.

Chocolate is another major dietary factor in heart disease. The chocolate that covers candy bars today consists of a "compound chocolate," in which cocoa butter and chocolate liquor—two expensive ingredients—are replaced by cocoa powder and vegetable fats. Many candy makers use hydrogenated soy oil, which is not at all the same thing as soy oil. Hydrogenated oil is oil that has had extra hydrogen ions added to it to change it from a liquid to a solid. When you add extra hydrogen ions to a food substance, you change its chemical configuration and then you do not have the evolutionary enzymes to digest it. Hydrogenated fats, found not only in chocolate but in margarine also, are a cause of atherosclerosis, the deposition of cholesterol in the lining of the arteries.

It is, of course, next to impossible to eat chocolate without sugar, and when the sugar changes your mineral relationships, some of the minerals become toxic. Toxic minerals cling to the cholesterol and cause hardening of the arteries. If you don't eat hydrogenated fats or sugar—which means you don't eat chocolate—and don't let the stress in your life become harmful, you will probably not get heart disease. Research suggests that it is just that easy.

Obesity

To some, it might seem silly even to discuss obesity and its relationship with sugar; the connection seems so obvious. Others might say that if I just eat 800 calories a day—regardless of whether they're from carbohydrates, fats, or proteins—I will lose weight. There are so many factors implicated in those 800 calories, however, that it is not reasonable to speak in those terms at all.

Reducing calories does reduce weight, but if you choose to eat 800 calories in candy bars, here is what else will happen. Sugar creates an artificial appetite which causes you to eat more and leads to obesity. The overuse of sugar can make your blood sugar yo-yo up and down, causing hunger pangs, shakes, perspiration, and other symptoms. Sugar will also cause you to become sensitive to certain foods and cause allergy-addiction. The cravings and hunger pangs that come with food allergies are certainly not conducive to dieting.

A computer is needed to calculate most diet regimes, and then, after all the mathematical exactitude, the program doesn't work. Calorie counting doesn't take into account how satisfied you are with what you put in your mouth. A four ounce candy bar is equivalent in calories to three pounds of beets or eight average apples, but doesn't go nearly so far in satisfying your appetite. Burning up the calories of a large apple requires nineteen minutes of brisk walking; burning off a candy bar takes twice that. Because sugar has no vitamins, minerals, enzymes, or fiber, it satisfies neither your hunger nor your body's needs.

We all have an "appestat" which should turn off when we have had enough calories. When thin people eat candy bars, their appestats tell them when they have had enough and they quit eating. When fat people eat candy bars, their appestats don't function correctly, and they don't know when they've had enough. They can't tell when they're full, so they keep eating. It seems to be a vicious cycle for overweight persons.

Sugar is implicated in a long chain of events in the body which lead to obesity. The minerals in the body become unbalanced, enzymes don't function correctly, food does not digest properly, and allergies occur. Allergies cause addiction, addiction causes cravings, and overeating is the result. So forget the 800 calories, and eliminate sugar and other refined foods—such as white flour, spaghetti, and pizza—from your diet if you want to lose weight. Get back to the basics: vegetables, legumes, protein, and do your exercise.

Candida Albicans

Candida albicans is an organism that lives in all of us. Babies have it and adults have it. It is a normal fungus which occupies space in the gastrointestinal tract, the genitourinary tract, and can get into the circulatory system. When our body chemistry is in harmony and our immune system is strong, candida lives happily within us. It might even do us some good; we don't know.

When the body is out of homeostasis and there are only six or so functioning units of calcium in the bloodstream rather than the usual ten, the cells become deficient and inefficient. The immune system can't handle candida when the cells aren't functioning correctly, and this fungus overgrows in the body. Diets rich in sugar can stimulate the fungal growth, as can birth control pills, antibiotics, cortisone, cortisonelike drugs, and immunosuppressant drugs used in cancer therapy and other therapies. These drugs kill off the good bacteria and leave space for the fungus to proliferate.

Dr. C. Orion Truss found out that when candida overgrows, it secretes an estrogen very much like the body's own estrogen. In fact, this estrogen can substitute for the body's estrogen. Candida's estrogen can occupy the binding sites of our cells so that regular estrogen can't get into the cells. Unfortunately candida's estrogen is only 1/100 percent as potent. If all the binding sites where you need estrogen to be functioning are filled with something that is 1/100 percent as potent, and you are already estrogen-starved, you are in trouble.

Candida overgrowth can cause other troubles as well. In its normal form, in the gut, candida is round. When it starts to overgrow and a large number of them appear, the candida enters the mycelia stage and grows roots that will penetrate the walls of the intestine. By the time the candida is overgrown, the tissue integrity of the bowel wall is compromised, and the wall becomes very weak. If you kill the root at this time, through the use of antifungal drugs or other aids, you will leave a hole in the intestinal wall through which undigested food can pass. The immune system will be unable to handle the food, and you will become allergic to it. As the body heals, so will the intestinal wall.

Symptoms of a candida problem include vaginal itching, burning, discharge, indigestion, bloating, and fatigue. We think we are victims of the candida, but we are not. We have to force the candida to overgrow inside of us; we have to feed it. Sugar is the main substance that feeds candida, and elimination of sugar is one of the main cures. But candida loves wine and all alcohol, and you might also watch out for yeast, mushrooms, aged cheese, nuts, seeds, and fruits. Since distress also upsets the body chemistry and suppresses the immune system, learning to deal with the distress in your life is most important for eliminating excess candida from your body.

Tooth Decay

The secretion of excess calcium is one clear sign of a mineral imbalance; tooth decay is another. Many clinicians believe that the first signs of the degenerative disease process are seen in the mouth. If you had many cavities as a child, chances are you will have many diseases as an adult—unless you stop upsetting your body chemistry.

Almost every tooth in my mouth is filled with gold, silver, or a composite. When I was a teenager, my parents felt that they could help me as an adult by having all of my fillings changed from amalgam (silver) to gold. For about four months I went to the dentist every Monday to have this work done. My dentist didn't believe in painkillers; he wanted to know when he was near the nerve, and my pain would let him know. I vividly remember dreading those Mondays.

Then, as an adult—until I stopped eating sugar—I had to go to the dentist every three months rather than the usual six because so much plaque would build up on my teeth. Between visits I would take a nail pick and scrape the back of my teeth to remove the excess plaque. Now that sugar is out of my diet, I see the dentist only once every six months, and there is little or no plaque on the back of my teeth.

Studies have shown a definite correlation between tooth decay and the amounts of calcium, magnesium, and phosphorus in the body. When the levels of these minerals in a group of volunteers were examined, the group with two or more dental cavities per year was found to have higher than normal calcium and magnesium levels in the blood, but lower than normal phosphorus levels, particularly in saliva. In this same study, 10 percent of those tested had adequate phosphorus levels in their saliva; this was reflected in a finding of one cavity or less per person, and most of the people in this category had no decay at all.

When the phosphorus level drops due to the ingestion of sugar, and the calcium/phosphorus ratio becomes unbalanced, it causes an acid state in the mouth. Acid is also formed when bacteria in the plaque on the teeth interact with sugar. Tooth enamel begins to dissolve at around pH 5.5; after the ingestion of sugar, the pH value on the surface of the teeth may go as low as 4.5. It remains low for about twenty minutes, then slowly returns to neutrality. The repeated consumption of sugar causes a continual production of acid and the maintenance of a low, or acidic, pH in the mouth. As with osteoporosis, it is clear that removing sugar and other substances which cause a calcium/phosphorus imbalance is a necessary step to stopping this degenerative disease.

Nevertheless, tooth decay continues to run rampant. Dentists tell us to brush more, to use dental floss, not to let babies fall asleep with bottles filled with milk or apple juice, to have fluoride treatments, and to use fluoride toothpaste. These suggestions assume that if sugar is not allowed to linger in the mouth, there is no danger of tooth decay. Anything that affects the teeth can't help but affect the rest of the body, and imbalances plaguing the body will affect the teeth as well.

When you are in homeostasis, your teeth are secreting mucus in a microscopic way. They are cleansing themselves. The glands in the soft tissues do the secreting and cleansing; the secretion comes out through the enamel rods of the teeth and keeps them from decaying. When you're not in homeostasis, when you're eating sugar, for example, something quite different happens.

Ralph Steinman, a researcher from Loma Linda University, put tubes down the throats of rats to bypass the teeth. He then gave the rats sugar water. Within a matter of minutes the fluid movement of the secretion was reversed. The mouth fluids started going through the enamel rods into the dentin. The bacteria by-products in the mouth are acidic; as long as the fluids are going out of the teeth, the acid from the bacteria doesn't decalcify the enamel. As soon as the fluids start going back into the teeth, decalcification starts in the bottom of the pits of the teeth. This suggests that at least part of tooth decay is due to a system malfunction, and not just a tooth surface problem.

While it's true that sugar starts in the mouth and that's where tooth decay occurs, this study seems to show that decay comes from unbalancing the body chemistry. Unless the body is thought of as a whole, instead of just a number of parts, the truly deleterious affects of sugar cannot be fully measured.

Multiple Sclerosis

Multiple sclerosis (MS) is a baffling disease of the nervous system for which medical science has few answers. I call it an allergy of the nervous system.

Other clinicians think the same way. Arthur Kaslow, M.D., found that many foods caused symptoms. Red meat, sugar, fruits, and flour products were frequent culprits. Yet different foods affected different people. Kaslow also found that foods that were tolerated in small quantities were not well tolerated in large quantities. He did not state that a person with MS has exhausted his enzyme systems due to imbalanced mineral relationships. Large amounts of any food cannot be tolerated by people with upset body chemistry. He concluded that small amounts of food eaten five or six times a day, minus the foods to which the patient reacts, is the best diet. I couldn't agree more. This is the best diet for all people who have symptoms. See Food Plan III in Chapter 8.

Inflammatory Bowel Disease

Inflammatory bowel disease has two major categories. The first one is ulcerative colitis, which only affects the inner lining of the colon. The second is Crohn's disease, which can irritate the deeper layers of the intestinal wall.

Any segment of the intestinal wall—twenty feet of small intestine and five feet of large intestine—is vulnerable to attack. Many other names are given to this disease depending on the area affected: regional enteritis, ileitis, colitis, granulomatous colitis, and ileo colitis.

Usual symptoms are diarrhea, weight loss, and cramping. Yet blood, urine, and stool tests as well as barium enemas show the person to be the owner of a normal bowel. Some patients show other symptoms not associated with the gastro-intestinal track such as hay fever, headaches, asthma, arthritis, and fatigue.

A variety of studies have shown that most people with inflammatory bowel disease can control their symptoms by eliminating foods to which they react. The foods most commonly sighted as being the problem are sugar, wheat, milk, corn, coffee, tea, and citrus fruits. The person must be aware that any food can cause symptoms; therefore, the person must be meticulous about testing for foods which cause the symptoms.

The best way to find the abusive foods is to withdraw all foods for twelve hours or until the pain has stopped. Then introduce one food at a time and watch for symptoms. Research from various sources shows that people formally afflicted can live symptom-free once they eliminate the foods causing the problems. The symptoms not associated with the gastrointestinal tract also disappear.

It is wise for people with inflammatory bowel disease to introduce acidophilus into their diet because their bowel has been stripped of healthy bacteria. Acidophilus will help bring it back.

Canker Sores

Studies from Australia show that canker sores can be eliminated by finding offending foods. Patients with recurring cankers of the tongue and mouth were unresponsive to treatment over periods of months. Twelve patients were then placed on a restricted diet for eight weeks. Half of the people had complete clearing of their cankers, which promptly reoccurred with food challenge. The offending foods identified in the study: dairy products, wheat, chocolate, tomato products, vinegar, citrus, and pineapple. The author does not say if the people who did not respond were allowed to eat sugar or other offending foods which could have upset their body chemistry again and made them allergic to other foods. I believe that if the patients had removed all abusive foods as well as foods that caused the cankers and not upset their body chemistry by stress or other factors, all twelve would have responded to treatment.

Gallstones

A recent article in the *British Medical Journal*, entitled "The Sweet Road to Gallstones," reported that refined sugar may be one of the major dietary risk factors in gallstone disease. Gallstones are composed of fats and calcium. Sugar can upset all of the minerals, and one of the minerals, calcium, can become toxic or nonfunctioning, depositing itself anywhere in the body, including the gallbladder.

One out of ten Americans has gallstones. This risk increases to one out of every five after age forty. Gallstones may go unnoticed or may cause pain—wrenching pain. Other symptoms might include bloating, belching, and intolerance to foods.

Cystic Fibrosis

The original medical descriptions of cystic fibrosis characterized it as a disease of the pancreas. The long-term survival, without correction of the basic problem, which is malabsorption, selenium deficiency, as well as other nutritional deficiencies, leads to lung disease and reduced immune status. Once a person becomes deficient in one mineral, then the functioning of the other minerals becomes impaired also. Therefore, the person becomes not only selenium-deficient but deficient in other minerals as well. Dr. Joel Wallach has been improving the health of cystic fibrosis patients by eliminating foods to which the person reacts, which gives the small intestine a chance to heal itself and allows increased absorption of selenium, zinc, protein, essential fatty acids, and other nutrients. This, in turn, allows the mineral-dependent pancreatic enzymes to function more readily; the food digests and the immune system is no longer bombarded with undigested food. Then the immune system can also function correctly.

We all have a genetic blueprint. A person who has cystic fibrosis has a genetic blueprint with a pancreas that does not function optimally. This person cannot upset his body chemistry in the slightest, or symptoms will manifest themselves saying all is not well. Again, take out the food, as well as other life-style factors that are upsetting the body chemistry, and just give the body a chance to heal. It will.

Future Generations

Changing your dietary habits can do more than help you avoid ailments like those listed here. If you are of childbearing age or younger, you have a chance to improve the genetic blueprint of your children.

All of us have from time to time noticed things about ourselves which we inherited from our parents—the color of our eyes, the shape of our nose, certain personality traits, and so on. It is also possible to inherit genetic strengths and weaknesses, particularly in the glands of the endocrine system, which will be with us for life. If we abuse our bodies over and over with sugar and other harmful substances, these inherited weaknesses may not be able to stand the stress of daily abuse, and the degenerative disease process may prevail. Even worse, the weaknesses we create in our bodies may be passed on to our own children.

An unbalanced body chemistry and weak endocrine system can be passed down over generations, with increasingly serious results. A man by the name of Francis Pottenger studied cats over several generations. He fed one group of cats a normal cat diet of raw foods; another group received the same foods, but after the foods had been cooked; and a third group was given the raw food diet accompanied by condensed milk, which contains sugar. The cats in the first group lived the longest and gave birth to healthy cats over two generations. The second group of cats did not live as long and gave birth to two generations of cats, each of which was less healthy than the former generations. Although all the cats were getting the same food with the same vitamins and minerals, cooking seemed to destroy some of the nutrients in the food.

Adding sugar to the diet made those nutrients less

available, as was shown by the deterioration over three generations of the third group of cats. These cats, who drank the condensed milk, gave birth to a second generation afflicted with many weaknesses, including hair that was not as shiny and thick as the first generation. The third generation was not able to reproduce and the litter died out.

Like these cats, each of us inherits an endocrine pattern from his or her parents, and we pass this pattern on to our children.

I recently took a trip to Egypt. Although most of the people would not be considered middle class by our standards, no one is starving. The Egyptian government subsidizes a healthful whole wheat bread, which we call pita bread. In many villages along the Nile, I observed primitive methods for making this bread, which consists solely of whole wheat flour and water. A twelve-inch-round pita cost one cent, so it was easily affordable and available to everyone.

At hotels along the way, however, I was served a breakfast of white toast, white croissants, white rolls, and jelly. Even when I asked for Egyptian bread at the hotels, most of the time I couldn't get it. On the streets I saw the people eating breakfasts of falafel (beans and pita bread) or pita bread stuffed with okra, lettuce, tomato, and small amounts of beef. In the hotels, where the clientele were more affluent, refined foods prevailed. When I returned to Cairo, what little pita bread I saw was made of white flour and was very expensive. There was no whole wheat flour in the bakeries of Cairo, and white flour had been used to make bread, cakes, and pastries.

The living conditions are still primitive in the villages in Egypt. The sanitary conditions are poor, and I'm sure that there are many deaths at birth and in infancy due to unsanitary conditions and communicable diseases. No doubt those living conditions will improve in the years to come, life expectancy will increase, and the favorite foods of the so-called advanced nations, sugar and white flour, will become more and more popular. As a result of this, the quality of those added years will be marred by arthritis, osteoporosis, cancer, heart disease, and other degenerative diseases. The endocrine systems of the villagers will be worn down, and the weaknesses will be passed on to future generations. Affluence seems synonymous with refined foods, cakes, pastries, tobacco, and other abusive substances. The more affluent people become, the further they stray from their native diet, and the weaker future generations become.

There is no way that you can change your own endocrine blueprint once you become an adult, but your life-style can make a difference in the way you feel now and in the future. The continual use of sugar, the use of other abusive foods, or the use of foods to which you are allergic depletes the endocrine glands' ability to function. When these glands are abused day in and day out, over a period of years and eventually through several generations, a certain degree of nonfunctioning and abnormal functioning of these overworked glands occurs.

Any disease state is the body protesting its life-style. I don't know why life needs to be so confusing when it seems so easy. Just take away from the body what it doesn't need and give to it what it does need and it will heal itself. In the next chapter we'll examine other substances—including alcohol, caffeine, and food additives—which, like sugar, must be avoided before the body can return itself to health.

6 | Sugar's Helpers

By now, it should be obvious that eliminating sugar from your diet is an essential step to keeping healthy and avoiding degenerative disease. Simply going without sugar is not enough. There are many other harmful substances which must be understood and avoided, substances such as alcohol, caffeine, rancid fats, aspirin, artificial sweeteners, food additives, and mercury.

Alcohol

Alcohol, like sugar, is absorbed very quickly into the bloodstream. The absorption process begins in the mouth and continues in the esophagus and stomach. Because alcoholic beverages are made up of various grains (such as wheat, rye, corn, or barley), the residue from these various grains also moves quickly into the bloodstream. Many people who drink become allergic to these grains. The repeated exposure to alcohol, in addition to the everyday use of grain in the diet, can exhaust the enzymes necessary to digest these residues. As discussed in Chapter 2, this causes undigested food to be absorbed into the bloodstream, with allergies as a result.

Alcohol that is not absorbed sooner reaches the large intestine and expands the cells of the intestinal lining. The alcohol, and any other food that happens to be in the intestine, can also be absorbed into the bloodstream without being completely digested. When alcohol is consumed with meals, then, there is a four times greater risk of allergic reaction than drinking alcohol alone. Alcohol has the same effect on the body as sugar—and if you're drinking alcohol with sugar (such as in a Manhattan or a gin and tonic), you are giving your body a doubly harmful dose.

Dr. George Ulett tested three groups of people—social drinkers, members of Alcoholics Anonymous, and active alcoholics—to see if alcoholics had more food allergies than other people. He found that alcoholics were, as suspected, reactive to more foods than the other two groups. Social drinkers had the second highest amount of reactions. The members of AA, who consumed no alcohol at all, had the least amount of food allergies. It seems obvious that alcohol is detrimental to the body's ability to digest and assimilate food properly; it would be wise to drink little, and when you do drink, drink alcohol without food.

When alcohol upsets our body chemistry, our digestive system suffers also. For example, there seems to be a connection between alcohol and hypoglycemia. Dr. William H. Philpott has found that 95 percent of all alcoholics are hypoglycemic. I interviewed a number of people at an Alcoholics Anonymous meeting, asking the same question each time: "Do you remember eating a lot of sugar as a child?" One person answered, "I can remember many times eating all the sugar in the sugar bowl." Another said that she couldn't remember eating large amounts of sugar, but she did drink five or six soft drinks a day. Many remembered eating sugar obsessively as part of their daily life in childhood.

Not all people who were sugarholics as children will grow up to be alcoholics, but there does seem to be a correlation between sugar addiction and alcohol addiction. Alcoholics Anonymous is a tremendous help to alcoholics with the psychological support and education they provide, but it is ironic that they also provide coffee, doughnuts, and other sweet foods at their meetings. These foods can suppress the immune system of nutritionally deficient people, such as alcoholics often are. Sugar can lower the blood sugar level and put these people in a hypoglycemic state—with all the symptoms of withdrawal and cravings for alcohol.

Studies also show that alcohol changes the body's ability to metabolize zinc. A person might be getting enough zinc in his or her diet, but if alcohol is also consumed, the cells are less capable of utilizing that zinc, and a deficiency results. This deficiency is seen as the principal cause of cirrhosis of the liver, a disease characterized by progressive destruction of liver cells and liver shrinkage. When moderate amounts of alcohol are ingested, there is an immediate decrease in the amount of zinc in the liver. As little as four alcoholic beverages a day over a period of time can cause liver damage.

Alcoholics get most of their calories from alcohol, rather than nutritious foods, so they are more than likely to have a nutrient deficiency. In addition, food absorbed too quickly through the alcohol-expanded walls of the small intestine cannot provide the body with whatever nutrients it might have. The intestinal mucosa doesn't have time to absorb vitamins and minerals, and it takes from months to years to recover these normal physiological capacities. A diet of only small amounts of protein, complex carbohydrates, and some fats, eaten in small amounts four or five times a day, supplemented with vitamins and minerals, is a good way to stop upsetting the body and letting it heal itself.

The link between sugar and alcohol can be most vividly

seen in an experiment conducted by Dr. Ruth Adams. Dr. Adams put laboratory rats on a "teenage" diet of coffee, doughnuts, hot dogs, soft drinks, apple pie, spaghetti and meatballs, green beans, white bread, and cake—primarily foods with hidden or not-so-hidden sugar. Eighty percent of the rats on this diet preferred to drink alcohol instead of water. In fact, they had a craving for alcohol. The other 20 percent preferred water that had been sweetened with the sugar equivalent of two cocktails. When half of the rats were put back on a diet of healthful food, the quantity of alcohol consumed fell. The rats who stayed on the poor diet continued to increase their consumption of alcohol until it reached one quart a day.

Clearly, sugar increases the craving for alcohol, and alcohol promotes the same kind of bodily harm as sugar. Other abusive substances, such as caffeine, can have the same effect.

Caffeine

Caffeine can actually increase the amount of sugar in the bloodstream. Caffeine stimulates the adrenal glands, which release adrenalinelike substances called catecholamines. These cause the heart to pump harder and the liver to release stored sugar. This sugar raises the blood sugar level, and the body's response is to prepare insulin in the pancreas to bring that level down to normal; this process, as we saw in Chapter 4, can result in the eventual exhaustion of the pancreas.

The release of sugar causes the "lift" most people associate with caffeine, but because caffeine throws the body chemistry out of balance, that lift is short-lived. The rush of insulin from the pancreas frequently goes so far beyond restoring normality that the sugar level falls below normal, causing extreme fatigue and other hypoglycemic symptoms. It may be hours before the body's chemistry returns to normal, and if another cup of coffee or tea has been ingested, the cycle of imbalance will continue.

Caffeine can cause other problems as well. There may be a connection between caffeine intake and birth defects, benign breast lumps, irregular heartbeats, and other serious medical problems. Caffeine stimulates the central nervous system and can be responsible for symptoms such as insomnia, nervousness, and anxiety. It's also a cardiac muscle stimulant, a diuretic, and a stimulant of gastric acid secretion in the stomach. In 1980 the FDA advised pregnant women to avoid or minimize the consumption of products containing caffeine.

Jeffrey Bland, Ph.D., the noted biochemist, can't say enough nasty things about coffee. His studies show, among other things, that caffeine elevates cholesterol levels in the blood. Bland also explains that the reason for the frequency of ulcers in coffee drinkers is that coffee stimulates the secretion of gastric juices.

Caffeine isn't the only element in coffee which plays havoc with the body. A study detailed in the Tufts University "Diet and Nutrition Letter" shows that coffee can inhibit iron absorption by 39 percent, or as much as 87 percent when coffee or tea is consumed with or up to one hour after a meal. (Drinking coffee or tea before the meal did not have the same effect.) One of the authors of the study, Dr. James D. Cook, claims that it isn't the caffeine that interferes with iron absorption, but a family of binding substances called polyphenols which are found in coffee. This group of chemicals strong-arms iron and escorts it out of the body. Since decaffeinated coffee also contains polyphenols, it too carries off needed iron. Herbal teas are not known to prevent iron absorption; therefore, they're good alternatives for those who want to give up coffee and regular forms of tea.

In spite of the known facts that coffee can cause

gastritis, heartburn, secretion of calcium in the urine, increased stomach acid and stomach discomfort, cystic breast conditions, and anxiety, the public continues to consume mountains of coffee beans, tea leaves, and cacao nuts. Dr. Eyi Takaahushi, of the Tohoku University School of Medicine, has found a correlation between the amount of coffee a country consumes and the number of deaths from cancer of the prostate. Other data indicate that it is the sugar used in coffee, rather than the coffee itself, which is the cause of prostate cancer; a definite correlation was also found between sugar consumption and cancer of the breast, ovaries, intestine, and rectum.

Specialty coffee stores, groceries, co-ops, and health food stores offer a variety of decaffeinated coffee beans that have been decaffeinated by the Swiss water method rather than the methylene chloride method.

In 1990, H. Robert Superko of Stanford University's Lipid Research Clinic reported that the blood levels of low density lipoproteins (LDL) increased an average of seven percent in one hundred eighty-one men who drank decaf coffee that had been deffeinated using the water method. Here is another good reason to start tasting herbal teas.

Drugs

It is well known that many drugs unbalance the body chemistry.

All drugs must be detoxified or undergo changes in the body before they can be eliminated. This detoxification usually goes on in the liver with the aid of enzymes, which are mineral-dependent. Unfortunately when a person needs drugs, the body chemistry is already upset and the minerals and enzymes are not functioning optimally. The drugs add an extra burden to the already compromised body. Cortisone, for example, raises the blood sugar to higher than normal levels. My research with urine calcium secretion shows that many antibiotics increase the calcium in the urine, thereby upsetting the body chemistry. Antacids, in addition to damaging the digestive system, can cause mineral imbalances and do damage to bones.

Most antacids that I have seen on the market contain aluminum. (One exception is Tums.) Antacids that contain aluminum, such as the popular stomach medications Mylanta and Maalox, cause a loss of calcium and phosphorus through the urine. However, since they don't produce any noticeable side effects, people continue to take them for stomach pains and indigestion.

These drugs work by binding and neutralizing gastric acid. Unfortunately they also bind with and prevent the absorption of phosphoric acid, which is then carried away in the stool. To compensate for this, the bones release some phosphorus into the bloodstream, along with the calcium with which it was bound. This calcium is quickly carried away by the kidneys.

Aluminum antacids, taken year after year, can deplete the skeleton of calcium and phosphorus, and cause thinning and weakness of all the bones. Then such minor incidents as tieing one's shoe or walking up the stairs can lead to bone fractures—a condition in which the bones crack but do not break completely—and the resulting stiffness, weakness, and pain are often mistaken for arthritis. Unfortunately it takes years for the cumulative bad effects of repeated doses of antacid to show up. Later in life, people tend to accept bone pain and fractures as a natural part of aging.

Antacids—with or without aluminum—also harm the bones by interfering with digestion. Calcium is absorbed in the upper part of the small intestine, and acid is essential to that process. Most antacids are used by people over forty years old, whose normal stomach acid has already decreased along with their calcium absorption. Although they take the antacid because of heartburn and the feeling that they are secreting too much acid, chances are they are not secreting enough of the kind of acid that helps in digestion: hydrochloric acid.

There is a simpler way to deal with problems like heartburn and indigestion, and that is to stop them from happening in the first place. Since caffeine stimulates the secretion of gastric juices, eliminate all caffeine from your diet. Don't eat so much at one meal that your digestive juices become exhausted, and remove all sugar from your diet. Dr. John Yudkin has studied acidity and digestive activity before and after sugar ingestion in healthy people. The results show that two weeks of a sugar-rich diet is enough to increase both stomach acidity and digestive activity of gastric juices—the kind one finds in people with gastric or duodenal ulcers. The sugar increased stomach acidity by 20 percent or so, and the enzyme activity was tripled.

Drugs such as thiazide diuretics increase the risk of magnesium inadequacy. These drugs also increase risk of heart disorders because they can cause abnormalities in glucose and lipid metabolism.

In addition to their other possibly dangerous effects, many drugs on the market today contain hidden cornstarch and lactose (a sugar found in milk). Although foods containing cornstarch and lactose must be labeled as such, no such law applies to drugs. In fact, the law in this case protects the drug companies. Trade Secrets legislation allows lactose and cornstarch to be labeled as "inert substances," and their presence may be concealed even from your doctor or pharmacist.

Drugs which contain both of these allergenic substances, cornstarch and lactose, include antifungal agents
such as nystatin as Mycostatin tabs (Squibb) and ketoconazole
as Nizoral tabs (Janssen); progesterone in the form of Provera
tabs (Upjohn); tranquilizers such as Valium tabs (Roche);
and corticosteroids including cortisone acetate tabs (Upjohn),
hydrocortisone tabs (Danbury, Purepac), prednisone tabs
(Phillips Roxane, Danbury, Purepac), dexamethasone (Philips
Roxane), dexamethasone as Decadron (Merck), and triam-
cinolone (Danbury).

Rancid Fats

Almost twenty-five years have elapsed since a report
stated that the breakdown product of charcoal-broiled beef-
steak causes cancer. The substance, benzo(a)pyrene, is
produced during the breakdown of fat that drips from the
steaks onto the hot coals. Smoke containing the benzo(a)pyrene
then collects on the surface of the meat. The formation of
these carcinogenic free radicals is dependent on the very
high temperature required for the breakdown of fat.

When fats are overheated, they can become rancid.
The natural process of oxidation in the body, which produces free radicals (atoms lacking at least one electron), is
made faster, much faster, when rancid fats are being oxidized. There are many different kinds of free radicals,
among them peroxide, hydroxyl group, and superoxide; and
all are poisonous. Enzymes such as peroxidase, catalase,
and superoxide dismutase are required to take the free
radicals and turn them back into useful products. As stated,
enzymes depend on minerals in order to function; when the
body's mineral balance is upset by rancid fats, enzymes are

unable to function correctly, and free radicals may be allowed to build up unimpeded.

If rancid fats continue to be consumed, the store of these enzymes may be exhausted altogether. The body will be unable to deal with free radicals normally, and the immune system must come to the rescue. It is best, therefore, not to overheat fats or to eat deep-fried food, particularly when body chemistry has already been unbalanced by sugar and other harmful substances.

Other Overcooked Foods

Many articles have been written that indicate that the eating of meat may give rise to certain forms of cancer of the digestive tract. A detailed study at the University of California at Berkeley concludes that it is not the meat itself that does the damage, but rather the way the meat is cooked. Meat that is cooked at high temperatures contains carcinogens. A recommended way of cooking meat is to do it slowly, as with a pot roast or in a Crockpot.

Fats are not the only food that can become less digestible to the body when overcooked. All protein, whether wheat protein or vegetable protein (meats, vegetables, and legumes all have protein in them), has the same chemical configuration. Over millions of years, our bodies have evolved enzymes that match up with protein molecules in our intestines. However, protein has a heat labile point—a temperature at which the protein becomes denatured and changes its configuration. Our enzymes are not designed to digest protein in this configuration. Noxious chemicals (those same free radicals) are produced, cross the intestinal membranes, enter the bloodstream, and then must be fought by the immune system. Researchers Barbara Schneeman and George Dunaif, of the University of California at Davis, concluded that, no matter how alluring they may seem, bread, milk, meat, eggs, and any other foods cooked to a golden brown have less food value than their counterparts.

Dr. Francis Pottenger, as discussed in Chapter 5, studied the effects of raw and cooked food on cats over a ten-year period. He was studying cat diseases when, quite by accident, he saw the effects of different diets on cats. Local restaurants had been supplying him with cooked meat scraps to feed the cats, but when the restaurants could not supply enough cooked meat, Pottener obtained raw meat from a wholesaler. He was surprised to see that the apparent health of the cats eating the raw meat contrasted with that of the ones who had been fed cooked meat. The cats fed raw food had good, shiny fur, produced healthy litters, and died of old age or injuries suffered in fighting. The cats who had eaten cooked food showed skeletal changes and were unable to reproduce efficiently. They showed signs of respiratory problems, food allergies, dental disturbances, and other health problems.

Pottenger found that the cats could be so reduced in vitality by just one year of a diet considered "adequate" for human consumption that they needed two or three years to recover—if they recovered at all. The same effect has been noted in laboratory rats. Rats were fed nonfat dry milk as their only source of protein for four weeks. One group of rats was given unheated milk; a second group ingested milk heated to a light brown at 121° C; and a third group drank milk heated, for forty-five minutes, to a cocoa brown.

The rats on the unheated milk thrived, grew, and gained weight. Those ingesting the light brown milk took ,in less food and lost weight, while those consuming the cocoa brown milk lost even more. The researchers discovered that browned proteins stayed longer in the stomach, indicating poor digestibility and poor absorption. As food gets darker, it changes its chemical configuration until our enzymes cannot digest it. A healthful diet for humans may consist of at least 50 percent raw foods, because these foods contain more of the vitamins, minerals, and enzymes so necessary for digestion and assimilation.

Aspirin

Although aspirin is not a food, many people ingest it as part of the daily diet. Doctors prescribe it for everything from headaches and menstrual problems to joint pains and heart disease. Indeed, there is evidence of aspirin's positive effects. One researcher found high levels of prostaglandins in infected chickens. When these chickens were fed aspirin, the prostaglandin levels went down and the mortality rate fell from 80 percent to 42 percent in two days. The aspirin clearly blocked the prostaglandins and improved the resistance to infection.

Yet agents such as aspirin, which inhibit one or more of the enzymes involved in prostaglandin synthesis, may cause negative alterations of body function. Another researcher, Dr. Edith Stanley, found that aspirin blocked an area of the immune system needed for the healing process. Aspirin was shown to keep the infection-fighting leukocytes from traveling to the inflammatory tissue. By suppressing the body's natural response to infection, aspirin may "relieve" the symptoms caused by the leukocytes battling the invading viruses, but the reproduction of the virus is left unchecked. These viruses are then free to spread within the body, prolonging and complicating the illness, if leukocytes continue to be hindered.

Researchers are finding that aspirin and other pain medication can cause irreversible damage to the kidneys and lead to kidney failure. It doesn't take very much. Just three regular aspirin a day, two kilograms in six years, can seriously impair the vital cleansing function of the kidneys. For those people living in hot climates or on low-salt diets the problem is even worse.

Dr. Stanley gave aspirin to a group of sick people and discovered that this group had 17 to 30 percent more viruses than a group treated with placebos. In addition, the amount of virus contained in the nasal discharge of the aspirin-treated volunteers was considerably higher than in those volunteers untreated with aspirin. Therefore, taking aspirin increases the threat of spreading illness to husbands, wives, children, and co-workers.

Leukocytes are not the only blood components adversely affected by aspirin; platelets, those cells in the blood which keep us from bleeding to death, are also disrupted. When a blood vessel ruptures, collagen tissue, which makes up the basement membrane of blood vessels, is exposed. The collagen signals the platelets to release a mineral substance, adenosine diphosphate, which makes the platelets sticky enough to bind together. Aspirin can destroy adenosine diphosphate and adhere itself to sticky platelets, making them incapable of binding to one another.

As few as one or two aspirin tablets can have this effect on the body, and platelets remain in this condition for about seven days—the life-span of each individual platelet. One ordinary dose of aspirin, then, can permanently destroy a platelet's ability to clump together with other platelets when necessary. Anyone who takes two aspirin tablets twice a day is maintaining a consistently ineffective platelet system and cutting down on the body's normal response to external injury. In addition, aspirin has been found to cause small amounts of internal bleeding in 60 to 70 percent of all people, regardless of the form of aspirin. The usual blood loss is a teaspoon or so; an occasional patient loses as much as three ounces.

A new study strongly links the use of aspirin by children and teenagers to Reye's syndrome. This ailment is marked by the sudden onset of vomiting, often with fever and sometimes accompanied by lethargy, severe headaches, and changes in behavior. These symptoms can progress quickly to convulsions, delirum, and coma. Reye's syndrome is fatal 20 to 30 percent of the time. Another study, conducted by the federal Centers for Disease Control, found that children suffering from flu or chicken pox were twelve to twenty-five times more likely to develop Reye's syndrome when given aspirin than sick children who did not take the drug. After a few days of protest, the drug industry decided to put warning labels on bottles of aspirin for children.

Of most importance in our study of the immune system and food allergies, however, is aspirin's destruction of the intestinal lining. When the gut lining is damaged, large food molecules are allowed to pass through; undigested protein enters the bloodstream, causing an immune reaction. Aspirin, like sugar and alcohol, can be a direct cause of food allergies. All in all, it is better to let the natural healing process progress on its own, without the help of aspirin.

Food Additives

The body's adaptive mechanism must cope with large amounts of synthetic chemicals in foods. It is estimated that the average individual ingests at least one gallon of synthetic additives, coloring agents, pesticides, and preservatives in a year's time. Dr. Lewis Mayron tested chemicals used as coloring agents for foods and found destruction of both red blood cells and antibodies by the tested chemicals in the blood.

In the 1970s there was a great deal of controversy about nitrates, the chemicals used to cure processed meats. Research has shown that nitrosamines, the product of nitrites and nitrates, when combined with the stomach's naturally produced hydrochloric acid, are potent animal carcinogens and are likely to cause cancer in humans as well. (Although some vegetables are high in nitrite, vegetables also contain ascorbic acid, which acts as an inhibitor of nitrosamine formation.)

In the past five years the federal government has attempted to lessen the public exposure to nitrites, nitrates, and nitrosamines. Levels of nitrites used in processed meats have been reduced, and, with a few exceptions, nitrate use in curing meats has been banned altogether. Nitrosamines in ham and bacon have been significantly reduced.

Here are a few steps you can take to further reduce your exposure to dangerous nitrosamines:

1. *Take vitamin C.* Since ascorbic acid is a proven inhibitor of the formation of nitrosamines, taking vitamin C whenever nitrites are consumed will help. Vitamin supplements, cabbage, peppers, lettuce, and potatoes are all good providers of vitamin C.

2. *Take vitamin E.* Research has indicated that naturally occurring vitamin E, found in cereals, grains, and vegetable fats, may also prevent the formation of nitrosamines.

3. *Eat meats that have not been cured with nitrites and nitrates.* Health food stores offer bacon, bologna, salami, hot dogs, and even hams that are chemical-free.

4. *Store and cook vegetables properly.* Cook only the quantity of vegetables you plan to eat. Don't leave vegetables at room temperature once they have been cooked, and don't keep leftovers for more than two days in the refrigerator.

Sweeteners

Many people, in an attempt to avoid sugar, turn to nonsugar sweeteners as substitutes, but these sweeteners can be equally harmful. Let me tell you a little about aspartame, a sweetener marketed under the trade name NutraSweet (NutraSweet is a trademark of G. D. Searle & Co.).

Aspartame is used in diet sodas and soft drinks, and is also packaged in small packets for table use in coffee, on cereal, and so on. Whereas table sugar is only about thirty-five cents a pound, aspartame costs thirty dollars a pound. This is due, in part, to the many studies done before the Food and Drug Administration would allow aspartame to be put on the market. As you read on you will find that more studies need to be done to ensure its safety.

Aspartame is made up of three different substances: phenylalanine, aspartic acid, and methanol (wood alcohol). When these components are digested, they are released into the bloodstream. It has been demonstrated that the effects of plasma and brain phenylalanine and tyrosine (both amino acids) are increased by aspartame in humans; high levels of these large amino acids in the brain can affect the synthesis of neurotransmitters and bodily functions controlled by the autonomic nervous system, such as blood pressure. Aspartame also inhibits the release of glucose into the bloodstream and induces the release of serotonin (an inhibitory transmitter) within the brain, which may affect behaviors such as sleep and hunger. Therefore, dieters may be only adding to their problems by drinking sodas with aspartame. Aspartic acid, when absorbed in excess, has caused endocrine disorders in mammals.

Methanol, a poisonous substance, is added during the

manufacturing of aspartame. When aspartame-sweetened diet drinks are used in hot weather and ingested during and after exercise to replace fluid, the intake of methanol can exceed 250 milligrams per day, or thirty-two times the Environmental Protection Agency's recommended limit of consumption for this toxin. The aspartame content of a liter of cola drink is approximately 555 milligrams and therefore 56 milligrams per liter of methanol. If a 60-pound child consumed two thirds of a two-liter bottle of cola drink, which could readily happen on a hot day, the child would be consuming over 732 milligrams of aspartame. This alone exceeds what the Food and Drug Administration considers the ninety-ninth percentile daily consumption level of aspartame. The child would also absorb over 70 milligrams of methanol from the soft drink, almost ten times the EPA's recommended daily limit of consumption for methanol.

The FDA, Dr. Richard Wurtman (professor of neuro-endocrine regulation at the Massachusetts Institute of Technology), and Woodrow C. Monte (director of the Food Science and Nutrition Laboratory, Arizona State University, Tempe, Arizona) have received well over a thousand complaints relative to aspartame consumption. The most common complaints and symptoms are dizziness, visual impairment, disorientation, ear buzzing, a high level of SGOT in the blood (an enzyme that breaks down protein into amino acids), tunnel vision, loss of equilibrium, severe muscle aches, numbing of extremities, inflammation of the pancreas, episodes of high blood pressure, and hemorrhaging of the eyes.

There have been very few studies of the long-term effects of this sweetener, and this nonfood should be used with great caution. This is also true of saccharin, a sweetener which has been around for quite a while and is banned in some countries including Canada. It is interesting to note that the only U.S. producer of saccharin is the Sherwin-Williams paint company, and that saccharin is made from petroleum products.

Studies indicate that saccharin causes cancer in test

animals. Instead of banning saccharin, the law requires warning labels on foods containing saccharin and a display of warning signs in establishments selling products containing the substance. With the choice between sugar, aspartame, and saccharin, the public would be better off if it just had its "sweet tooth" extracted. As the White Queen said in *Alice in Wonderland,* "The rule is, jam tomorrow and jam yesterday—but never jam today."

Mercury

Mercury poisoning from amalgam (silver) fillings can be the cause of symptoms ranging from fatigue and nausea to headaches and double vision. One third of hypersensitive people with amalgam fillings will run a subnormal body temperature, as low as 96 or 97° F. Mercury hypersensitivity can also be indicated by a metallic taste in the mouth and excessive saliva. Mercury poisoning can deplete the body's store of such minerals as lithium, which is used today to treat depression.

Interestingly enough, dentists appear to be particularly susceptible to mercury poisoning. Dr. DeWayne Ashmead, a biochemist and nutritionist, accidentally noticed high mercury levels in hundreds of dentists he was testing for other minerals. At an annual meeting the American Dental Association sampled dentists' urine and found ten percent of dentists to be suffering from excessively high mercury levels. Perhaps due to the lithium depletion caused by mercury poisoning, dentists have a high divorce rate among professional groups and a rather high suicide rate. Bringing the body back into balance can alleviate many of these symptoms. Removing the mercury toxicity from the mouth can help stop the unbalancing.

*   *   *

Other substances and environmental stimuli can become dangerous when the body chemistry is unbalanced by sugar. Once sugar had slowly but surely taken its toll on my immune system, many substances with which I had lived in harmony for a lifetime became troublesome. I didn't change my neighborhood, home, or habits, but many things I had lived with before became intolerable. I would go to my parents' boat and have allergy symptoms from the dampness and mold. Whenever the winds came up, the pollens in the air would cause watery eyes and sneezing. The dog I had loved and petted in the past suddenly made my throat and ears itch when I hugged him. While filling my car with gas, I found the fumes gave me a feeling of fatigue. The perfume I had worn for years began to make me feel slightly nauseated. Reading the newspaper made me fall asleep. Did I ever think that the world was conspiring against me! Instead, it was my own dietary choices and my abusive life-style that created a condition in my body which allowed environmental substances to upset my chemistry even more.

My unbalanced body chemistry and compromised immune system were the causes of each of my new maladies. Only by removing sugar and other harmful substances from my life did I return to homeostasis and normalcy. Many people today become universal reactors—apparent victims of the twentieth century. However, far from being victims, they are creators of their own destabilized bodies by their wrong choices over a lifetime. They can change their condition just as I did.

In the next chapter we'll discuss another factor which must be dealt with before homeostasis can be maintained—stress.

7 | Stress

Stress is a trendy word today. It makes for great conversation at cocktail parties. You can read about it week after week in books on the best-seller list, or call in and talk about it on radio shows. Psychologists, psychoanalysts, psychotherapists, hypnotherapists, accupressurists, and anyone else with a point of view make daily appearances on TV shows to help us deal with the stress in our lives. Weekend seminars on stress abound—not just in California, where such activity has been popular for many years—but all over the United States.

Although the word *stress* is commonly used, *distress* might be a better word. The concept of stress as a demanding life event is too imprecise to be used as a measurement of how stress affects health. What one person considers stressful another might find stimulating. How a person responds to life events, not the events themselves, influences susceptibility to disease. Adequate coping with a high-stress life may reflect a psychological hardness which is actually protective. Failure to cope well with stress, on the other hand, can impair a person's ability to fight off illness.

Psychological Stress

Distress has been found to have virtually the same effect on the body as sugar. It unbalances the calcium/phosphorus ratio, causing a rise in calcium and a decrease in phosphorus; it can also cause calcium to drop and phosphorus to rise. Whenever minerals change their relation to one another, the body goes out of homeostasis, enzymes do not work, food does not digest, and the immune system must go into action.

When I did my research on the effect of sugar on the calcium/phosphorus ratio, I also did research on stress. I drew blood from the arms of two volunteers to determine their normal calcium/phosphorus ratio. I then had each of them immerse one hand in ice water for one minute. This is very stressful to the body; one volunteer immediately experienced back pain which she hadn't felt in years. Afterward, I took another blood sample to check the calcium/phosphorus ratio. In one volunteer the calcium went up and the phosphorus dropped. In the other the opposite happened: the phosphorus went up and the calcium dropped. Of course, in both cases the ratio changed.

This research indicates how instantly distress can change the body chemistry. Other research has examined the long-term consequences of distress on the immune system. Researchers at the Albert Einstein College of Medicine compared crises in the lives of children with minor ailments to crises in children with cancer. In the year before the cancer patients became ill, they had suffered twice as many crises in their lives as the other children. They had undergone such emotional upsets as parents' separation, death in the family, and change of school. In a different study the emotional histories of thirty-three children suffering from leukemia were examined. Researchers found that thirty-one had experienced a traumatic emotional loss or move within two years before the leukemia was diagnosed. Half of these upheavals had occurred only six months before.

The connection between distress and disease can be seen in adults as well. Dr. Lawrence LeShan, a New York City psychologist, studied 450 adult cancer patients and found that an incredible 72 percent had been frustrated, lonely, and had experienced a major emotional loss anywhere from six months to eight years before the cancer was diagnosed. By comparison, Dr. LeShan found that only 10 percent of a control group of cancer-free people had a similar emotional pattern. In another study Dr. Steven Schleifer, a psychiatrist at New York's Mount Sinai School of Medicine, and his colleagues found a significant decline in the activities of the white blood cells of a spouse during the first two months after the loss of a loved one. The cells continued to be suppressed for one year.

Dr. Margaret Linn and her colleagues at the Veterans Administration Medical Center in Miami, Florida, conducted a study of heavy smokers. Dr. Linn found no difference between the number of stressful events—marriage problems, business problems, or deaths—in the lives of heavy smokers with cancer and those without cancer. She did find that those smokers who developed cancer perceived these events as being negative and felt more guilt about them than did those who did not develop cancer. Questions asked in this study were general enough so that this difference was apparently present before the cancer group became ill.

Sugar and Psychological Stress

Recently my daughter was in the hospital for minor surgery. After her operation the doctor put her on a liquid diet. I was in her room one night when a nurse brought her dinner: Jell-O, ice cream, grape juice with corn sweetener, and tea with two packets of sugar. I was told by the dietician that this liquid diet had been approved by a large committee of doctors and was used in hospitals all over the Los Angeles area. I assume that those children who had cancer were probably being given ice cream, Jell-O, and other sweet foods while they were in the hospital, since sugar seems to be the mainstay of hospital diets. Between the stress caused by the hospital stay and the sugar, their little bodies didn't have a chance.

Like sugar, distress changes the mineral relationships in the body, and also exhausts the endocrine glands. It is the endocrine system which takes the initial beating when the body is under stress. When we are challenged, for example, the adrenals secrete adrenaline, triggering a rise in blood pressure and increased blood flow to muscles and the brain. A continued adrenal stimulus can exhaust these glands. Since adrenaline also stimulates the liver to convert its glycogen (stored sugar) into glucose (blood sugar), the pancreas has to secrete insulin to convert the glucose into energy in the cells.

Constant stimulation and increased metabolic rate help deplete the biochemicals that go into the production of hormones, the glands' chemical messengers. Certain individuals, due to genetic weakness or poor diet, may experience a hypoglycemic response. Excess insulin circulating in the bloodstream lowers the blood sugar, depriving the brain of its principal fuel. The pancreas, which is particularly vulnerable to overwork, can eventually lose some or all of its insulin-producing capability, and diabetes may result.

The correlation between stress, sugar, and the endocrine glands can be clearly seen in a study from the Soviet Union conducted by Dr. I. I. Brekhman. Dr. Brekhman stressed 246 female white rats by hanging them for eighteen hours by the fold of skin on the back of their necks. This stress produced several marked biochemical changes. The sugar content of the blood increased from 86 milligrams to 128 milligrams per milliliter. There was an increased discharge of hormones into the blood, as well as a reduction in the amount of glycogen (stored sugar) in the liver.

Before the rats were stressed, both the experimental and the control groups had a stress index of zero.* When the experimental rats were stressed, their index rose to seven. When these same rats were fed white sugar, the stress index increased to nine. If we relate this result to humans, we can see that an individual can get an overload of stress from various sources. He or she might be under distress, eat a candy bar, drink a cup of coffee, and inhale hazardous chemicals. One stressor at a time might have been safely handled, but when they attack the body collectively, it doesn't have a chance.

How to Handle Stress

It is important to limit these stressors as much as possible. A divorce, loss of a job, high mortgage payments, trouble with in-laws—all these are life events which affect us emotionally to such an extent that they may make us physically ill. Just as stressful emotions can make us sick, positive emotions can help to keep our body in balance and often offset the damage of distress. There's a lot of evidence that positive emotions such as love, faith, humor, and a positive mental attitude can help protect us against a variety of diseases.

How we bring joy into our own lives can vary from person to person, but we must make sure that there are

---

*Unfortunately the authors did not clearly define the stress index.

people we love in our lives. Try to express love every day, and be open and honest about your feelings. Have fun, watch funny movies, or read funny books, and you'll be helping your body chemistry and promoting good health.

Distress certainly played an important role in the disease process in my body. From the time I was very young, I had to be the best at whatever I did. I was the one who had to collect the most newspapers in the newspaper drive. It wasn't enough to be a United States Junior Tennis Champion; I had to be the fastest runner in every class at school as well. Becoming president of each class became an obsession for me. My drive to excel was relentless.

This drive to excel, this need to be the best, was just a substitute for my self-esteem. I needed all those outside achievements in order to feel good about myself. Finally, in my thirties, with the help of psychoanalysis, I learned to accept and love myself. I realized that I didn't have to win a tennis tournament before people would be my friends. I didn't have to excel at anything. People were my friends just because they liked me.

The first thing that changed because of my analysis was the way I played tennis. I didn't play any better, but it became so much easier. My body just seemed to flow. It felt so good. No one was looking over my shoulder anymore and asking, "What's the score?" No one was doing that before, either, but I had imposed that on myself in my drive to be or do better.

You have seen how there are many ways to upset the body's chemical balance. The next chapter will give you plans to use to help you change your life-style and regain or maintain health.

8 | A Practical Life Plan for Attaining and Maintaining Good Health

It is paradoxical that in a time of accelerating technology, of material abundance, of extended life-span, and of a supposed well-being, growing numbers of Americans are experiencing more and varied forms of health breakdowns. One out of two persons today is developing cardiovascular disease; one out of three, cancer; one out of five, diagnosable mental illness; and one out of five, diabetes. Birth defects are on the rise, and recent studies reveal that our children aren't as strong as children of fifty years ago. Scholastic scores continue to fall. New and unprecedented forms of disease are occurring. Allergies and low-energy conditions abound. The cost for health care (which is really disease care) is now a staggering three billion dollars a day.

Clearly, the quality of health is decreasing, and an increasing number of people are not responding well, or in a lasting way, to say nothing of long-range improvement, to appropriate medical care. Our "ignorant" ancestors, by contrast, had stronger bodies and a less material life-style. It is possible for people today not only to escape the perils of the modern life-style but also to avoid the downward spiral of degenerative disease. This chapter is devoted to showing a way based upon the principles we have discussed.

In the preceding chapters you have seen how sugar, other substances, and stress disturb your chemistry and can lead to degenerative disease. Now you will learn how damage can be reversed. Once you've licked the sugar habit and started following the plan given here, you'll be able to rebuild your enzymes, endocrine system, immune system, and, in fact, your whole body.

To regain and/or maintain good health, you must understand and act upon the following principles.

1. Disease and health result from the condition of the body's chemistry. Health breakdowns result from unbalanced body chemistry (a body whose minerals are out of the right relationship).

2. Your chemistry may unbalance quickly. Depending on your adaptive abilities, your chemistry may stay unbalanced or rebalance just as quickly.

3. The extent of any health breakdown is determined by the degree and duration of unbalanced body chemistry.

4. The only difference between a well person and a person with health breakdowns is that the well person can efficiently rebalance his or her body chemistry.

5. You are in control of your body's balance, through conscious and unconscious choices.

6. How your body responds to appropriate medical care, after a health breakdown, depends on the balance of your body's chemistry.

7. Through education and intelligent choices, you can increase conscious control of your body's chemical balance.

Four Arenas

There are four "arenas" in which we act and produce basic effects on our chemical balance. Let's take a closer look at what each arena involves, and the steps we can take to improve life-styles.

ELECTROCHEMICAL BALANCE

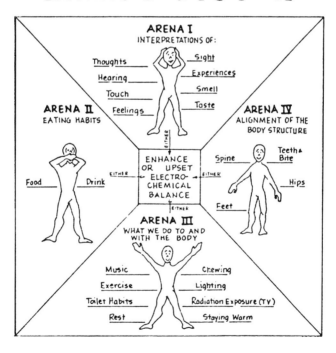

ARENA I: The Choices We Make in Interpreting What We and Others Do, Think, and Say

The mind can get in the way of health. Emotions we feel, good or bad, can change our mineral relationships and chemical balance.

It is important to observe the language we use and pay attention to the ways in which what we say, think, and do upset body chemistry. Once a decision is made to change a harmful life-style, we must commit to that action. Telling a loved one or a friend about the action is helpful. When it is difficult to follow through, it may be necessary to get some help from a therapist. As individuals we must find out why our conscious and subconscious are working against us. When body chemistry is upset by an abusive life-style, it is often difficult to follow through with commitments, because the mind is out of balance as well as the body.

ARENA II: The Choices We Make in Deciding What to Eat

Arena II deals with the foods, inhalants, and drugs that we ingest. There are foods which upset the body chemistry and foods which enhance it. This book has dealt particularly with upsetting foods. Beginning on page 110, there are three detailed plans which will help you choose foods which are good for you.

As a former sugarholic and chocoholic, I remember the pleasure (misdirected, as I know now) that I had from eating sugar. I'm not sure how, when, where, or why it happened, but that thought process has changed. Now I think in terms of eating foods that don't upset my body chemistry. I enjoy my food just as much as formerly, and possibly more. I certainly can eat more, because I've given up all those refined foods with so little bulk and so many calories. You can do the same.

ARENA III: The Choices We Make in Deciding What to Do with and to Our Bodies

Arena III deals with body mechanics and stimuli external to the body.

Body mechanics include chewing, toilet habits, and exercise. With good habits you can help bring your body back into alignment. Follow these guidelines:

1. Chew each bite of food at least twenty times. Digestion begins in the mouth; an enzyme in saliva starts the process. Help your digestive system by chewing well.

2. When nature calls—answer. If you wait a half hour, nature may no longer call. The body wants to get rid of waste. When undigested food stays in the colon too long, it can become toxic. The immune system then has to deal with the by-products of putrefaction.

3. Drink enough water to stay hydrated. Drink water between meals.

4. Do some form of exercise that uses opposite arm-leg movements. This includes running, swimming, walking, or anything where your arms swing back and forth in a balancing motion. If you do aerobic exercise, all the better. If you don't, then deep-breathe to get air as far into the lungs as possible. Begin your exercise with stretching.

5. Don't sleep within three feet of an electrical outlet or wire *that is in use.* Wires *in use* radiate an electromagnetic field.

6. Sit at least ten feet away from the television set when watching.

7. Don't work under fluorescent lighting. Sitting under fluorescent lighting all day can exhaust the body. A full-spectrum light can be bought at many health food stores today and used in place of conventional fluorescent lighting.

8. Studies show that hard-rock music can change the body chemistry. Listen to music that does not upset the chemical balance of the body.

9. Assure yourself six hours of quiet sleep per night, and sleep warm.

ARENA IV: The Choices We Make Regarding Alignment of the Body Structure

A body out of alignment, whether jaws, cranium, spine, hips, or feet, will experience distress. Distress, in turn, upsets mineral relationships. Arena IV is easy to deal with if the other three arenas are in balance. A chiropractor makes an adjustment, and it will hold because there is good protein digestion and tissue integrity. If you are not functioning well in other arenas, and mineral relationships have been upset, tissue integrity will be compromised. A chiropractor may make an adjustment, but it won't hold. The four arenas are inter-related; each must be balanced before health can be achieved.

Extended Application of the Four Arenas

This book is not intended as a handbook or manual in response to all ailments. It should be useful to most people most of the time. Its concepts provide the basis for a response to any disease no matter how serious. Certainly no one will ever be harmed by removing sugar, fat cooked at high temperatures, and other abusive food from his or her diet. The extent to which these concepts must be applied depends on one's genetic blueprint, for how long and severely one's body has been abused, and the nature of the resulting condition.

Recent research on AIDS shows that an approach similar to the one outlined in this book has been used to improve the immune system and the general condition of AIDS patients. Patients using this approach used a variety of methods dealing with all four arenas. Arena I activity included ongoing support groups, psychotherapy, maintaining a personal journal, relaxation training such as meditation, biofeedback or self-hypnosis, daily practice of the Simonton Visualization Method (read *Getting Well Again*) and philosophy/religion inquiry. Arena II activity included Food Plan III, minus foods to which a person reacts, supplemented by megadoses of vitamins, minerals and herbal preparations. Arena III and IV activity included saunas to cleanse and detoxify, massage, Hatha Yoga, aerobic exercise, homeopathic remedies, colonics, chiropractic adjustment, the Alexander Method, and Rolfing.

Each of us is a unique individual and each responds differently to a variety of therapies. For some people simple modifications in life-style can greatly improve their health. Other people need to explore many different modalities in order to give the body a chance to heal.

A Test to Determine Homeostasis in Your Body

This is an easy method for determining your calcium/phosphorus ratio. It is possible to find which arenas are giving you trouble, which foods most unbalance your body chemistry, and how well you are maintaining your health. A simple test tells you if you are secreting too much calcium, too little calcium, or a normal amount of calcium. This test works by measuring the amount of calcium in the urine.

Since calcium works only in relation to phosphorus, this test tells whether the phosphorus is too high for the calcium present (no calcium will show up in the urine), whether the phosphorus is too low for the calcium present (too much calcium will show up in the urine), or there is a correct amount of calcium for the phosphorus present (there will be a normal amount of calcium in the urine).

Although the test detects only calcium, if the calcium/phosphorus ratio is out of balance, the rest of the minerals in the body are also out of balance. When the calcium/phosphorus ratio is in balance, the rest of the minerals are in balance, and the body is in a state of balance. This home kit for monitoring your electrochemical balance comes with a booklet which explains its use. The booklet is written by Nancy Appleton and Dr. Bruce Pacetti. The kit can be obtained from:

> Nancy Appleton, Ph.D.
> P.O. Box 3083
> Santa Monica, CA 90403-3083

See order form on page 162.

Food Plans

The following food plans are effective particularly when used in conjunction with the kit.

CAUTION: Following Food Plans I, II, or III may initiate withdrawal symptoms and a phenomenon called physiological and psychological detox. You may experience different symptoms, many similar to withdrawal from any addiction. Fever, depression, headaches, chills, and fatigue are the most common symptoms.

Food Plan I

1. Avoid all foods in Categories IV and V (see food lists starting on page 112). Eat any other food.

2. If after being on this plan for seven days, you are not feeling better, your body chemistry requires a more comprehensive food plan. Therefore, proceed with Food Plan II.

Food Plan II

1. Avoid all foods in Categories III, IV, and V, and eat foods in Category II only in small amounts and only between meals. For meals, eat Category I foods.

2. If after being on Plan II for seven days, you are still not experiencing better health, you need to proceed to Food Plan III.

Food Plan III

It is clear that your unbalanced body chemistry involves more than just the foods common to body chemistry upset.

Food Plan III is designed to provide complete nutrients to your body in their most bio-available form. Adherence to this plan automatically handles some complex food-related biochemical problems which Food Plans I and II did not handle. The procedures and foods of Food Plan III are the least stressful to your body chemistry.

1. For the next fourteen days eat only foods from Category I. Eat one small portion from each food group four or five times a day. Remember to follow the Health-Promoting Eating Habits beginning on page 117.

2. If after fourteen days you are still not experiencing relief of symptoms and have addressed all four arenas, you'll need to see a qualified practitioner who can give you blood tests and a test for food sensitivities, and can help you to find foods that do not upset your body chemistry.

Food Categories

Category I

When prepared and eaten in a proper manner, the foods of Category I are tolerated best by the already unbalanced body chemistry of people with health breakdowns.

Group 1
GREEN LEAFY VEGETABLES

Artichoke
Brussels sprouts
Cabbage
Kale
Lettuce (all)
Spinach

Group 3
YELLOW/WHITE VEGETABLES

Cauliflower
Corn
Cucumber
Squash (all)

Group 5
ORANGE/PURPLE/RED VEGETABLES

Beet
Carrot
Eggplant
Pumpkin
Sweet potato
Tomato

Group 2
GREEN VEGETABLES

Alfalfa
Asparagus
Avocado
Broccoli
Celery
Chinese pea
Okra

Group 4
ROOT VEGETABLES

Jicama
Onion
Parsnip
Potato
Radish
Rutabaga
Turnip

HERBS/CONDIMENTS

Arrowroot
Basil
Bay leaf
Black pepper
Butter
Caraway
Chili pepper
Chive
Cilantro
Dill
Garlic
Ginger
Horseradish
Lemon
Lime
Mustard
Nutmeg
Olive oil
Oregano
Parsley
Rose hip
Rosemary
Safflower oil
Sage
Sesame oil
Sunflower oil
Tarragon
Thyme

Group 6

FISH	MEAT/ POULTRY
Anchovy	Bacon
Bass	Beef
Catfish	Chicken
Clam	Chicken egg
Cod	Duck
Crab	Frog's leg
Flounder	Lamb
Haddock	Liver, beef
Halibut	Liver, chicken
Mackerel	Pheasant
Oyster	Pork
Perch	Turkey
Red snapper	Venison
Salmon	
Sardine	
Scallop	
Shark	
Shrimp	
Sole	
Swordfish	
Trout	
Tuna	
Any other fish	

Group 7

BEANS/GRAINS

Azuki bean
Barley
Bean sprout
Black bean
Black-eyed pea
Buckwheat
Garbanzo bean
Green pea
Kidney bean
Lentil
Lima bean
Millet
Navy bean
Oat
Pinto bean
Red bean
Rice, brown
Rice, white
Rice, wild
Rye
Soybean
Split pea
String bean
White bean

If you are a vegetarian, use our Food Plans, but eliminate Group 6 and combine your beans and grains in Group 7 to give complete protein.

Category II

Certain areas of some people's body chemistry have become sensitive to these otherwise wholesome foods.

FRUITS	NUTS/SEEDS	HERBS/ CONDIMENTS
Apple	Almond	Allspice
Apricot	Brazil nut	Anise seed
Avocado	Chestnut	Chicory
Banana	Flax seed	Clove
Cantaloupe	Hazelnut	Cream of tartar
Coconut	Hickory nut	Paprika
Cranberry	Macadamia nut	Spearmint
Date	Pecan	
Fig	Pistachio	
Grape	Poppy seed	
Guava	Safflower seed	
Melon (all)	Sunflower seed	
Nectarine	Walnut	
Papaya		
Peach		
Pear		
Pineapple		
Plum (prune)		
Raspberry		
Strawberry		
Watermelon		

Category III

Overcooking, overeating, and eating with sugar have turned these normally well-tolerated foods into potentially abusive foods. These foods can now unbalance the chemistry of those who have already impaired their ability to rebalance their body chemistry.

YEAST	HERBS	MISCELLANEOUS
Baker's yeast	Curry	Carob
Brewer's yeast	Peppermint	Cinnamon
Mushrooms	Salt	Coffee
	Vanilla	Coffee, decaf.
		Cola bean
GRAINS	DAIRY	Corn gluten
Wheat bran	Blue cheese	Cornstarch
Wheat germ	Buttermilk	Fructose
White flour	Cheese (all)	Honey
Whole wheat	Cottage cheese	Hops
	Cow's milk	Molasses
FRUITS	Cream cheese	Tea
Grapefruit	Whey	
Mango	Yogurt	
Orange		
Tangerine	NUTS/SEEDS	
	Cashew	
	Peanut	

Category IV

These foods are always abusive to human body chemistry. Only those who remain adaptive can rebalance their body chemistry after frequent exposure to Category IV foods. The more Category IV foods consumed, the more rapid the deterioration in the body chemistry.

Alcohol	Cocoa	Malt
Beet sugar	Corn sugar	Maple sugar
Cane sugar	Corn syrup	Saccharin

Category V

These chemicals have known unbalancing effects on the body chemistry, and it serves your health to use them seldom and with caution.

Aspirin	Food coloring	Tobacco
Baking powder	Formaldehyde	Tylenol
BHT	MSG	Sodium benzoate
Caffeine	Petroleum by-products	

Simple Suggestions for Breakfasts and Snacks

People who are on Food Plan III, and eat only Category I foods, sometimes have difficulty with ideas for breakfast. Here are a few suggestions, many of which can also be used for snacks.

1. Potatoes: Cook potatoes the night before and refrigerate. In the morning slice potatoes and sauté in butter at a low temperature.

2. Baked potato with butter, guacamole, or pureed beans.

3. Corn tortilla with butter, tomatoes, an egg, and/or guacamole.

4. Oatmeal with butter.

5. Cream of Rice with butter.

6. Rice cakes with sliced avocado, tomato, onion, green pepper, or cucumber.

7. One egg omelet with sliced tomato, cut-up potato, green pepper, onion, or other vegetables.

8. One egg ranchero with corn tortilla.

9. Cooked rice with butter.

10. Steamed sweet potato with butter. Sweet potatoes are also good cold. They taste like candy.

11. One cup of popped corn.

12. My favorite quick breakfast is leftover rice heated with grated carrots, frozen peas, frozen lima beans, and butter.

Health-Promoting Eating Habits

Regardless of which Food Plan you're on, be sure to observe the following general health-promoting eating habits:

1. Chew each mouthful of food at least twenty times.

2. Do not wash foods down with liquids.

3. If you drink liquids during the meal, take small sips, and only when there is no food in your mouth.

4. Drink most of your liquids between meals.

5. Consume portion sizes you feel you can safely digest.

6. If you are emotionally upset or disturbed, eat smaller portions and chew more.

7. Do not overcook your food.

8. At each meal consume as much raw food as you do cooked.

9. Rather than eating large meals less often, consume smaller meals more often.

10. Examine each meal and snack from the viewpoint "Does any part of this meal upset my body chemistry?"

These suggestions will lessen the body chemistry insult from your food habits and facilitate a more efficient digestion, assimilation, and utilization of nutrients. In addition, you will be supporting your body's ability to rebalance its chemistry after other life-style insults. Finally, your response to appropriate medical care will be enhanced.

9 | Self-Help Techniques

By now you have a good idea of what both sugar and stress do to the homeostasis of the body and how they lead to the degenerative disease process. I hope that you have made a commitment to improve your diet and life-style and follow the Life Plan described in Chapter 8. Nevertheless, if you have been a sugarholic, you may still find it difficult to lick the sugar habit entirely. The following suggestions will ease you through those withdrawal periods when you have cravings but are trying not to eat sugar.

1. *Don't keep sugary food in your home.* Throw away any foods which contain sugar; pitch them right out. Then, if you need a "fix," you will have to drive to the store to feed your habit. This will give you time to think, and maybe you'll change your mind. If not, buy only enough to satisfy your craving. Don't buy any more than you can eat at the moment. Buy the smallest size of whatever it is you crave, and throw out what you don't eat. Better wasted outside the body than inside.

2. *Leave corn out of your diet.* Since so much of

the sugar in processed foods comes from a corn base, I suggest you leave corn out of your diet until you have given up sugar for two months. If you've been eating a lot of sugar, you're probably allergic to corn. Any form of corn—cornstarch, corn sweetener, corn bread, corn on the cob—could bring on a craving. In fact, any form of food to which you are allergic could cause a craving. Also avoid foods to which you know you are allergic.

3. *Use carbohydrates to battle hypoglycemia.* If you should go into a hypoglycemic state, with symptoms such as fatigue, perspiration, dizziness, light-headedness, or fainting, you may be tempted to eat sugar, thinking that this will bring your blood sugar level back to normal. Remember that this will help you only for the moment and will hurt you in the long run. An influx of sugar may lift the blood sugar level so high that it has to come crashing down again. What you need instead are complex carbohydrates such as potatoes, whole wheat bread, crackers, or even nuts. It will take longer for your blood sugar level to return to normal, but you'll avoid the yo-yo effect.

4. *Use healthy food for snacking.* Fast foods don't have to be unhealthful. I suggest that you steam three or four potatoes, sweet potatoes, yams, squash, and other foods containing complex carbohydrates and keep them in your refrigerator along with raw foods such as green and red peppers, jicama, carrots, and celery. Then, when you have a snack attack, you will immediately have food there that you can eat.

5. *Always read labels.* If there are any words that you cannot pronounce or spell on the label, don't put the food in your mouth. Also watch out for any words that mean the same as sugar. Ingredients must be listed on the label by their predominance, but don't be fooled by a product that lists corn sweetener as the third ingredient, invert sugar as the fourth, and dextrose as the fifth. This is a deceptive method of dealing with a lot of sugar in a package. If these three ingredients were combined on the ingredients list (and maybe they should be because all of them are *sugar*), there might very well be a greater amount of sugar in the product than of the first ingredient on the label.

6. *Eat protein in small portions.* Protein is absorbed and simultaneously broken down into amino acids. This makes possible the release of glycogen (sugar stored in the liver), the main function of which is to raise the blood glucose level. If the blood sugar level is raised, it must come down, and as the level falls, you may crave sweets. Next time you get a sugar craving, think about what you ate at your last meal; if there was a large portion of meat or fish, you might try cutting down on the portion. The body needs protein, but eat small portions at each meal, rather than a large portion at one meal. Some forms of protein may trigger cravings while others do not. This is another good time to get in touch with your body and the signals it's giving you.

7. *Taste sugar if you have to, but don't swallow it.* Another idea might be to put sugar, in whatever form, into your mouth, chew it, and then spit it out. This gives you the taste, but very little gets into the bloodstream. The best part is that you will be consciously rejecting the sugar by spitting it out.

8. *Get help from your friends.* Try going on the buddy system with a friend who's cutting out sugar, or just trying to reduce. Phone your buddy when you need a little support or before you go to the store for candy. Having to be responsible to someone else might put a slight guilt trip on you, and you might not be as likely to cheat. Besides, having support from a friend always feels good, whether it's for help or just for friendship. If you're craving sugar because of loneliness or depression, telephoning a friend will help that state of mind too. If you're a person who needs to be scolded, then pick someone who will do that. On the other hand, if all you need is support and someone who will listen, pick someone who will do just that.

9. *Exercise!* Exercising shuts down the appestat, that mechanism in the brain which controls appetite. Most people are not hungry after vigorous exercise. So exercise helps a person stay thin not only because it eats up calories but also because it cuts down on appetite. You can get double duty out of your exercise, then, if you wait until you have those cravings before you do your daily workout.

10. *Avoid artificial sweeteners.* If you give a rat saccharin, its body will be fooled into thinking it is sugar and will produce a boost of insulin. This could be part of the reason that artificial sweeteners are poor aids for weight watchers and sugarholics. I'm afraid that artificial sweeteners are not good substitutes for sugar. If worse comes to worst, many health food stores carry candies sweetened with maltose, sorbitol, or other forms of complex natural sugars, sugars which need some form of digesting and breaking down into simple sugars in the body. Choose these over artificial sweeteners such as saccharin and NutraSweet, and certainly over sugar. Table sugar, white sugar, needs little processing in the body. It gets into the bloodstream quickly— too quickly.

11. *Substitute carob for chocolate.* There are many carob candies on the market today, but I cannot recommend these, even if they are not made with sugar. All the ones I have seen contain hydrogenated fat, which is difficult for the body to utilize, as discussed on page 65.

You might use powdered carob, butter, and almonds, coconut, vanilla, or other ingredients to make your own candies.

12. *Set realistic goals.* You may not be able to cut out sugar all at once; phasing it out slowly is sometimes a better plan. Set a quit date, a deadline of when you want to stop eating sugar altogether. Each day, decrease your sugar intake by a given amount. If you slip, observe it but don't wallow—move on. Set your goal again. Realize that even one day without sugar is a triumph. When you finally do make your goal, reward yourself. Get yourself a massage, take yourself out to dinner, or do for yourself whatever feels good.

13. *Avoid temptation.* There are certain situations when you are more likely to eat sugar, and you should avoid these situations whenever possible. This doesn't mean you should quit your job, but you might change where you eat lunch, or take a walk when the fast-food truck comes.

14. *Use delaying tactics.* When you have a sugar craving, try to put off eating sugar for a half hour, then an hour. Substitute positive activities. Relaxation techniques work for some people; others use meditation.

15. *Take glutamic acid.* The amino acid L-glutamine (glutamic acid) has two major functions in the body. First, it fuels the brain—a feat matched by only one other compound, glucose. Second, glutamic acid restores hypoglycemic patients in insulin coma to consciousness at a lower blood sugar level than when glucose alone is used. L-glutamine might work for your sugar cravings. Take 500 milligrams three times a day.

16. *Avoid soft drinks.* A glass of mineral water with lemon, lime, or a tablespoon of orange or apple juice makes a great soft-drink substitute. Sugar-free soft drinks are not substitutes; the phosphoric acid in all soft drinks changes the calcium/phosphorus ratio.

17. *Brush your teeth.* Try brushing your teeth when you have a sugar craving. There is a little sugar in toothpaste, but not enough to do you any harm.

18. *Keep your body in homeostasis.* It may take awhile for your body to get back to homeostasis. Different organs can become oversensitive or underactive because of sugar. It will take time for the organs to reorganize themselves. You can help by avoiding any foods to which you are allergic and staying away from stressful situations. I recommend that you not eat fruit until you stop having cravings, because fruit has fructose and glucose in it, and it will raise your blood sugar. For a sugar-sensitive person, fruit can change the mineral relationships. Coffee is another no-no. Coffee can lower your blood sugar, and you might get such symptoms of hypoglycemia as dizziness, faintness, and perspiration, which could trigger off a sugar craze. Alcohol is a stimulant to some and a depressant to others. Avoid any stimulant or depressant. The foods that help keep the body in homeostasis are vegetables, legumes, and small amounts of protein.

19. *Be aware of psychological factors.* When you reach for that candy bar or soft drink, take a look at your life and its stressors. What events in your life make you crave sugar? When do you want to put something in your mouth to soothe yourself? Make a connection between what is going on outside of you and what is happening in your head. Try to break the cycle.

As your eating habits change, so will your taste buds. A carrot will seem as sweet as a candy used to. Lightly steamed carrots with a small amount of butter are now a delicacy to me when before they were something my mother made me eat. You will be pleasantly surprised how healthful foods taste much more sweet than they did before. Pages 126–137 contain health-giving recipes which will help you forget the absence of sugar in your diet.

10 | Epilogue

You have seen how eating excess sugar and abusing your body through other habits can jeopardize your health by upsetting your body chemistry. The minerals become deficient in the body. Since enzymes are dependent on minerals to function, the enzymes won't function as well, and therefore the food does not digest completely. Undigested food gets into the bloodstream. It can't be utilized by the cells to get the nutrients it needs in this undigested form. Our immune system must come to our defense and escort this foreign protein (the undigested food) out of the body. The immune system was not meant to do this continually, and the immune system is made of protein, which it is not getting because the protein is not digesting completely. When we do this over and over, we exhaust our immune system. The exhaustion of the immune system is the degenerative disease process. It depends on the genetic blueprint of the individual as to what disease will occur, arthritis, cancer, or other diseases that suppress the immune system.

I hope this knowledge is as useful to you as it is to me. It is exciting to me to feel that I know how to maintain my health and also to help others. I wonder how my life might be if I had had this knowledge twenty years ago or, better yet, as I was growing up.

I was born with an endocrine system that secreted less than the ideal amount of some hormones and more of others. In itself this would probably not have interfered with my quality of health or life. However, because of the stress I placed upon myself to excel as a child, and the incredible amount of sugar I consumed, my body became less able to cope with abuse. Twenty years of my adult life were plagued with health problems.

Today I am in better health than I have been since I was eighteen years old. I need less sleep (six and a half hours instead of eight and a half), have less fatigue, can play tennis two hours a day and not get tired, weigh my ideal weight, can consume an incredible amount of food, wake up happy, and go to bed happy every day.

Now that I have taken responsibility for my health, I am not a victim of the twentieth-century life-style. I eat well, in spite of all the processed foods in the markets; I don't let stress become distress; I treat my body well; and I get help when needed. I feel in control of my life and health. Control can be yours also.

Recipes

Soups

GARBURE

1 cup dried navy or pea
  beans, soaked overnight
8 cups water
2 potatoes, sliced
2 onions, sliced
1–2 leeks, sliced
2 medium turnips, sliced
2 carrots, sliced
½ cup dried split peas
1 bay leaf
1 teaspoon thyme
1 teaspoon marjoram
¼ cup minced fresh parsley
3 cloves garlic, minced
1 hot chili pepper
½ small cabbage, shredded
½–1 pound roasted pork,
chicken, goose, duck, beef,
or other meat (optional)

Drain the beans and set
aside. Bring the water to a
boil in a large soup pot. Add
the beans and all remaining
ingredients except the cabbage and meat. Cover and
bring quickly to a boil again.
Reduce heat and simmer for
1 hour. Add the cabbage and
roasted meat. Cover and bring
quickly to a boil once more,
then reduce heat and simmer
for 30 minutes. Discard the
bay leaf and chili pepper.
Remove the meat, slice it,
and place a serving in each
bowl. Add soup. Serves 4–6.

HOT ASPARAGUS SOUP

3 pounds asparagus, fresh or frozen
¼ pound butter
1 onion, chopped
6 cups chicken broth
½ teaspoon ground nutmeg
Salt and pepper
2 tablespoons chopped parsley or watercress

If using fresh asparagus, wash and snap off tough ends. Slice into 2-inch pieces. Heat butter in a large, heavy saucepan. Add onion and cook until tender. Cut off and set aside asparagus tips and add sliced asparagus stalks to onions. Cook 1 minute. Add broth and nutmeg. Season to taste with salt and pepper. Bring to simmer and cook until stalks are tender, about 18 minutes.

Add tips and cook until tender, about 3 minutes. Spoon out and reserve some cooked tips for garnish. Puree remaining cooked asparagus in a blender 2 cups at a time. Soup may be refrigerated at this point. To serve, reheat and serve hot, garnished with parsley and warmed, reserved asparagus tips. Makes 8 servings.

GINGERY CHICKEN SOUP

1½ pounds chicken breasts
6 cups water
1½ teaspoons salt
3 tablespoons grated, peeled ginger root
3 green onions, sliced diagonally
1 cup sliced mushrooms (optional)
1 (8½-ounce) can water chestnuts, drained and diced
1 teaspoon soy sauce
1 cup shredded lettuce

Combine chicken, water, salt, and ginger in a large saucepan. Bring to boil, reduce heat, cover, and simmer about 30 minutes or until chicken is tender. Remove from heat. Remove chicken and cool slightly. Strain broth and return to saucepan. Skim fat if necessary. Skin and bone chicken. Cut into ½-inch cubes. Bring broth to simmer. Add chicken, green onions, mushrooms, water chestnuts, and soy sauce. Simmer 10 minutes. Stir in lettuce just before serving. Makes 6 servings.

VEGETABLE CHOWDER

1 tablespoon safflower oil
1 medium onion, sliced
½ cup thinly sliced celery
1 clove garlic, minced
3 cups chicken broth
1 (16-ounce) can undrained
  tomatoes, chopped
1 cup sliced carrot
1 teaspoon dried basil leaves
¼ teaspoon black pepper
1½ cups garbanzos
1½ cups whole kernel corn
¼ pound zucchini, sliced (1
  cup)

Heat oil over medium heat in 5-quart pot. Add onion, celery, and garlic. Cook, stirring constantly, 5 minutes or until tender. Add broth, tomatoes, carrots, basil, and pepper. Cook about 25 minutes or until vegetables are tender. Add garbanzos, corn, and zucchini and cook 5 more minutes. Makes 8 servings.

MANHATTAN CLAM CHOWDER, MEXICAN STYLE

2 tablespoons oil or butter
½ cup diced onion
½ cup diced celery
2 tablespoons arrowroot
1 cup chicken broth
1 (12-ounce) jar green chile
  salsa
½ cup diced potatoes
1 tablespoon minced parsley
Dash thyme
1 tablespoon basil, crushed
½ bay leaf
Garlic powder
Salt and pepper
1 (6-ounce) can chopped
  clams

Heat oil in saucepan over low heat. Sauté onion and celery until transparent. Stir in arrowroot and cook over low heat 2 minutes. Add chicken broth and simmer 3 minutes. Add salsa, potatoes, parsley, thyme, basil, bay leaf, and garlic powder to taste. Season to taste with salt and pepper. Simmer until potatoes are tender. Add clams and simmer additional 5 minutes. Makes about 4 servings.

BROCCOLI SOUP with VEGETABLES

1 cup broccoli florets
1½ cups strong chicken stock
½ cup water (from broccoli)
½ cup corn kernels, fresh or
  frozen

1 medium tomato, seeded
Freshly ground pepper
Dash lemon juice

Steam broccoli florets in a small amount of water just until they are bright green. Remove the basket and add 1½ cups chicken stock to the water in the pan, which should be about ½ cup. Add the corn to this stock and water mixture and simmer for 5 minutes, or until corn is almost tender. Cut the tomato in thin wedges and add to the corn and stock. Chop and add the broccoli florets. Cook 5 minutes more. Add pepper and lemon juice. Makes 4 servings.

HEARTY BEET BORSCHT

3 large onions, chopped
3 beets, peeled and grated
1 carrot, chopped
2 potatoes, peeled and cubed
1 medium head red cabbage, shredded
2 quarts vegetable broth
2 cups fresh tomatoes, chopped and skinned
½ teaspoon dill
2 bay leaves, crumbled
1 tablespoon arrowroot
Salt

Combine all ingredients except salt in pan. Simmer for 25 minutes. Salt to taste. Makes 6 servings.

BOHEMIAN SPICED TOMATO SOUP

2 tablespoons butter
1 medium onion, chopped
2 stalks celery, chopped
2 quarts tomatoes, fresh, frozen, or canned
1 quart well-flavored vegetable stock
Salt and pepper
1 tablespoon (or more) mixed pickling spice, put in a stainless-steel tea ball

In a large kettle melt butter and sauté onion and celery until soft, but not browned. Add the tomatoes, stock, and salt and pepper. Bring to a boil. Be sure there are some pieces of bay leaf, chili pepper, ginger, and peppercorns in the pickling spice. Drop the spices into the soup and simmer for 1 hour or until the tomatoes have cooked to a puree and the soup smells marvelous. Makes 8 servings.

HOT BORSCHT (Blender)

Combine in a blender:
1 cup tomato juice
1 cup beets, peeled and diced
1 parsnip, diced
2 cups potatoes, diced
1½ cups white cabbage, diced
  Water if necessary

Blend until smooth. Sauté 2 minced garlic cloves in 1 tablespoon oil. Add blender mixture, a touch of vinegar, and cook for 20 minutes. Season with salt, pepper, paprika, and dill to taste. Pour into soup bowls, and top with parsley. Makes 4 servings.

Vegetables

FRESH POTATO MELANGE

¼ cup butter or margarine
2 large white rose potatoes, peeled and cut in julienne strips (about 3½ cups)
1 large onion, chopped (1 cup)
1 large carrot, thinly sliced (¾ cup)
2 ribs celery, sliced (1 cup)
1 clove garlic, chopped
2 cups chicken broth

1 bay leaf
¼ teaspoon dried leaf thyme, crumbled
¼ teaspoon salt
⅛ teaspoon pepper

In large skillet melt butter; sauté potatoes, onion, carrot, celery, and garlic 2 to 3 minutes, stirring occasionally. Stir in broth, bay leaf, thyme, salt, and pepper. Bring to a boil, cover, reduce heat, and simmer 10 minutes. Uncover, stir, and cook 5 minutes longer. With slotted spoon remove vegetables to serving bowl; keep warm. Reduce cooking liquid over high heat until slightly thickened, about 2 minutes. Pour over vegetables. Makes 4 servings.

PEPPERS STUFFED with BARLEY and CORN

4 medium green peppers
¾ cup cooked barley
½ cup cooked corn
1 large scallion, chopped
2 tablespoons parsley, chopped
  Freshly ground pepper
  Dash salt
½ teaspoon dried basil
½ teaspoon chili powder
1 large tomato, juiced and chopped

Wash peppers and cut off tops. Remove seeds and membranes and steam for 5–6 minutes. Cool. To make the filling, combine the barley and corn with the scallion, parsley, and seasonings. Wash the tomato and cut it in half crosswise. Juice it by running a spoon down into the seed "compartments" and removing the juice and seeds. Chop the tomato and add it to the corn and barley. Stuff peppers with mixture and place in oiled casserole pan. Pour a half inch of water, stock, or tomato juice in the bottom of the pan. Bake at 350 degrees, covered, for 15 minutes. Remove cover and bake for 10 minutes more, adding more liquid if necessary. Makes 4 small servings.

CURRIED PEPPERS and GARBANZOS

1 tablespoon butter
1 clove garlic
¼ cup sweet onion or scallion, chopped
1 medium green pepper, sliced thin
Sprinkle of freshly ground pepper
½ teaspoon dried basil
½ tablespoon chili powder
Dash each cumin, coriander, dry mustard
1 cup vegetable juice cocktail
¾ cup cooked garbanzos

Heat butter in a medium-sized skillet. Mince the garlic very fine and sauté it and the onion and green pepper in the butter over medium-low heat until the vegetables are beginning to turn soft. Do not brown the garlic or pepper. Season with freshly ground pepper and the rest of the spices. Do not add salt because the vegetable juice cocktail has enough in it already. Add the vegetable juice cocktail and cook for about 5 minutes to blend the flavors. Add the cooked garbanzos and heat through. If mixture seems too thin, mash a few garbanzos with the back of a fork and blend in to thicken. Makes 4 small servings.

SAVORY PEPPER PILAF

2 tablespoons butter
1 tablespoon safflower oil
1 clove garlic, minced
½ cup sweet onion, chopped
½ cup green pepper, chopped
(cont. next page)

1 cup cooked brown rice
Salt and pepper
1 tablespoon Worcestershire
    sauce

In a large skillet heat 1 tablespoon butter and the oil together. Sauté the garlic, onion, and green pepper in it until they are just beginning to turn soft and still crunchy. Add 1 more tablespoon butter and the rice to the skillet. Season with salt and pepper to taste. Stir the rice in with the vegetables until rice is heated through. Add the Worcestershire sauce and stir thoroughly. Cook 15 minutes. Makes 4 servings.

RATATOUILLE

4 cloves garlic, finely chopped
1 large onion, chopped
¼ cup olive oil
2 medium green peppers
2 zucchini, cubed
2 yellow squash, cubed
1 bunch parsley, chopped
4 tomatoes, chunked
1 bay leaf
1 teaspoon basil
1 teaspoon marjoram
¼ teaspoon oregano
2 teaspoons sea salt
Pepper to taste
8 large, firm, ripe tomatoes,
    blended to puree

Sauté garlic and onion in olive oil. Add cut vegetables and seasonings, then add tomato puree. Simmer until all vegetables are a little tender, not mushy. Serve over your favorite whole grain. Makes 6 servings.

VEGETARIAN STEW

1 tablespoon butter
2 cups fresh mushrooms,
    sliced thickly (optional)
¼ cup chopped onion
1 clove garlic, finely minced
3–4 medium tomatoes
1 medium zucchini, sliced
2 green peppers, seeded and
    cut into 1-inch chunks
½ teaspoon sweet basil
½ teaspoon marjoram
1 tablespoon finely chopped
    fresh parsley
Salt and pepper to taste
¼ cup white wine (optional)

In a large saucepan melt butter and sauté mushrooms, onion, and garlic till tender. Add vegetables and seasonings. Simmer, covered, till vegetables are tender, about 15 minutes. Add wine and continue to simmer another 5 minutes. Makes 4 servings.

LENTIL TOMATO LOAF

2 cups cooked lentils
2 cups canned tomato sauce
½ cup chopped onion
½ cup chopped celery
¾ cups oats
½ teaspoon garlic powder
¼ teaspoon Italian seasoning
¼ teaspoon celery seeds
½ teaspoon salt
¼ teaspoon pepper

Combine all ingredients in a large bowl. Pack into an oiled 9 × 5-inch loaf pan. Bake at 350 degrees for 45 minutes. Let cool slightly before unmolding. Makes 10 servings.

CABBAGE SCRAMBLE

½ cup tomato juice
½ teaspoon oregano
4 cups shredded cabbage
3 carrots, shredded
1 large onion, sliced and separated into rings

Place all ingredients in a large skillet or pot, in the order listed. Cover and simmer over low heat 10 minutes, stirring often. Remove lid, turn up heat, and toss until liquid is reduced. Serve hot. Makes 4–6 servings.

Meat Dishes

IRISH STEW*

1 cup water
¾ cup cubed lamb (2-inch cubes)
½ cup sliced potato
½ cup sliced carrot
¾ cup sliced onion
½ cup green beans, chopped
1 clove garlic, minced
1 small bay leaf
¾ cup sliced celery
¼ teaspoon dried rosemary
½ teaspoon dried mint
¼ teaspoon dried marjoram
2 tablespoons arrowroot

Bring ½ cup water to a boil over medium heat. Add lamb, vegetables, and herbs, lower heat, and cook until meat is tender. Mix arrowroot with ½ cup water and turn heat back up to medium. Move vegetables to sides of pan and stir arrowroot into broth. Continue to stir until sauce is thickened. Turn off heat and stir vegetables gently into sauce. Remove bay leaf. Makes 2 servings.

*Irish Stew comes from *The Candida Albicans Yeast-Free Cookbook*, permission granted by the author, Pat Connolly and Associates of the Price-Pottenger Nutrition Foundation, P.O. Box 2614, La Mesa, California.

SPANISH-STYLE RICE and GROUND BEEF

2 medium onions, diced
1 medium green pepper, diced
¾ pound ground beef
2 cups cooked brown rice
2 tablespoons safflower oil
3 tomatoes, chopped
2 tablespoons lemon juice
½ cup tomato juice
½ teaspoon pepper
1 tablespoon onion powder
⅛ teaspoon garlic powder

Saute onion, green pepper, ground beef, and rice in oil at low temperature until just lightly cooked. Add all other ingredients. Simmer 15 minutes. Makes 4 servings.

PERSIAN LAMB and BEAN STEW with HERBS

⅔ cup dried red kidney beans, white kidney beans (cannellini), great northern, or navy beans
7 cups water
2 pounds lean lamb, cut into 1-inch cubes
Salt to taste, if desired
Freshly ground pepper to taste
2 bunches, about ⅓ pound, fresh parsley
1 pound fresh spinach in bulk
5 tablespoons butter

1 cup finely chopped leeks
¼ cup finely chopped green onions or scallions
1 tablespoon finely minced garlic
5 tablespoons olive oil
2 tablespoons ground turmeric
2½ cups fresh or canned chicken broth
¼ cup fresh lemon juice

Put the beans in a bowl and add water until the beans are covered by about 2 inches of liquid. Let soak overnight and drain. (If the beans are labeled "no soaking necessary," skip this step.) Put the beans in a kettle and add the 7 cups of water. Bring to a boil. Cover and cook until the beans are tender, anywhere from 30 minutes to 2 hours, depending on the type of bean selected. Do not overcook. When the beans are tender, remove from the heat and drain them. Set aside.

Meanwhile, sprinkle the meat with salt and pepper and set aside.

Rinse the parsley and spinach and pat dry. Remove and discard any tough stems. Chop parsley and spinach coarsely.

Heat 3 tablespoons of the butter in a kettle and add the parsley, spinach, leeks, dill, green onions, and garlic. Cook, stirring, until the greens are wilted. Set aside.

Heat the oil and remaining 2 tablespoons of butter in a skillet and cook the cubed meat, a few pieces at a time, until it is browned. Do not crowd the cubes or they will not brown properly. As the pieces are cooked, transfer them to the kettle. When the last batch of cubes is browned, sprinkle with turmeric and stir briefly. Transfer this last batch to the kettle.

Add the chicken broth to the skillet in which the meat was cooked. Add this liquid to the kettle. Add the lemon juice and bring to a boil. Cover and cook about 1 hour or until the meat is almost fork-tender. Add the drained beans to the stew. Add salt and pepper to taste and stir. Continue simmering about 10–15 minutes. Makes 8 servings.

Salads and Salad Dressings

BULGARIAN BEAN SALAD

2 cups cooked navy beans or kidney beans
1 small green pepper, chopped
1 small sweet onion, chopped
1 large carrot, grated
¼ small head cabbage, shredded
2 tomatoes, chopped
Dressing:
    1 clove garlic, minced
    2 tablespoons chopped parsley
    Salt and pepper to taste
    ½ cup oil
    ¼ cup lemon juice

In a large bowl combine beans and remaining vegetables. Make dressing and pour over salad, tossing to coat thoroughly. Chill in refrigerator for 1 hour to blend flavors. Serve on romaine lettuce.

BASIC MAYONNAISE

2 eggs
1 teaspoon sea salt
¼ teaspoon dry mustard
4 tablespoons lemon juice
1¼ cups safflower oil (oil must be at room temperature)

Blend everything except oil. Add oil very slowly to egg mixture. Blend until thick. Will keep 1 week in refrigerator.

VEGETABLE RICE SALAD

4 cups cold cooked brown rice
1 cup sprouts
1 small zucchini (about 6 ounces), minced
½ cup scallions, minced
1 small green pepper, minced
4 tablespoons minced parsley
Dressing:
    ¼ cup lemon juice
    ⅓ cup oil
    Dash cayenne

Toss the rice with the sprouts, zucchini, scallion, pepper, and parsley. Mix the dressing ingredients and toss with the rice mixture. Chill.

MOLDED CHICKEN SALAD

3 cups cooked rice
2 cups chopped cooked chicken
1 cup cooked green peas
1 cup chopped celery
½ cup thinly sliced green onion including tops
1 avocado
¼ cup chopped pimiento
2 envelopes unflavored gelatin
½ cup double-strength chicken broth (cold)
⅔ cup mayonnaise
1 tablespoon lemon juice
2 teaspoons salt
1 teaspoon seasoned pepper

In a large mixing bowl combine rice, chicken, peas, celery, onion, avocado, and pimiento. Soften gelatin in broth; heat to dissolve. Combine with mayonnaise, lemon juice, salt, and pepper. Add to rice mixture and mix thoroughly. Spoon into a 1½-quart mold or individual molds. Chill until set. Unmold onto salad greens, if desired. Makes 6–8 servings.

BROCCOLI and POTATOES VINAIGRETTE

2 medium light-skinned potatoes
1 small head broccoli, separated into florets (about
1½ cups)
Dressing:
1 clove garlic
Salt and pepper to taste
2 tablespoons lemon juice
1 tablespoon water
2 tablespoons chopped parsley

Cut potatoes into large cubes, skins on. Steam until they are half done when pierced with a knife. Add the broccoli florets. Steam with potatoes until broccoli is just cooked and potatoes are cooked all the way through. To prepare the dressing, mince garlic rather fine. Add a little salt and mash the salt into the garlic until a paste is formed. Place in a cup and add pepper and lemon juice. Stir all this together. Add the water and taste the dressing. If it is too sour, add more water. Pour the dressing over the vegetables. Sprinkle with fresh parsley and serve warm. Serves 4.

PEPPER SLAW

1 large green pepper, sliced
paper-thin
2 cups white cabbage, shredded
1 scallion, sliced paper-thin
Dressing:
1 small clove garlic
¼ teaspoon salt
Freshly ground pepper
Dash dried basil
3 tablespoons lemon juice
4 tablespoons safflower oil

Wash vegetables, slice, and toss. To make dressing, mince and mash the garlic with the salt until it is a paste. Combine with other seasonings and the lemon juice. Beat in the oil with a fork. The dressing will begin to look cloudy and thicken slightly. Pour the dressing over the vegetables and either serve at once or chill. Serves 4.

Glossary

acute: rapid; short; sudden; severe

adrenal gland: one of two glands in the upper back part of the abdomen which produce and secrete vital hormones

adrenal medulla: the central portion of the adrenal gland, responsible for production and secretion of adrenaline

adrenaline (epinephrine): one of the hormones secreted by the adrenal glands

allergen (antigen): a foreign protein, as in a food, bacteria, or virus, that stimulates a specific immune response when introduced into the body

amino acid: the end product of protein metabolism

anterior pituitary gland: the front portion of the pituitary gland located at the base of the skull; it produces important hormones such as growth hormone

antibody: a substance produced in the blood, capable of producing immunity to a specific germ or virus; our bodies also form antibodies to undigested food in the bloodstream

antigen: *see* allergen

biochemistry: the chemistry of live tissue

body chemistry: the functioning of the body systems which depends upon the body's chemical balance, which depends upon balanced mineral relationships

carcinogen: any substance that causes cancer

cardiovascular: relating to the heart and blood vessels

cataract: a cloudiness in the lens of the eye which reduces the amount of light going through

cholesterol: a chemical component of animal oils and fats

chronic: pertaining to a disease of long duration

chymotrypsin: an enzyme found in the small intestine which aids in the digestion of proteins

clinical ecologist: one who looks for various causes of sickness which include maladaptive reactions, physical, mental, emotional, or otherwise, occurring on exposure to any substance, be it food, manufactured chemical, or pollutant

complement: a complex group of enzymes in normal blood serum that work together with antibodies; when complement is activated by antibody, it presents a serious threat not only to microorganisms but also to the host's own cells

cytotoxic: toxic to the cell

cytotoxic test: a blood test for food allergies

degeneration: deterioration of tissue with loss of function, eventual destruction of particular tissue cells

diabetes (mellitus): a chronic disease characterized by an excess of sugar in blood and urine

endocrine gland: a gland, such as pituitary, thyroid, and adrenal, which secretes its hormones into the bloodstream

enzyme: a protein that accelerates specific chemical reactions but does not itself undergo any change during the reaction; a biochemical catalyst; digestive enzymes are produced by glands and organs to break down complex carbohydrates into simple sugars, fats or lipids into fatty acids, glycerol, and glycerides, and protein into amino acids

epinephrine: *see* adrenaline

estrogens: a group of steroid hormones which are formed in ovary, placenta, testes, and possibly the adrenal cortex; besides stimulation of secondary sexual characteristics, they also exert systemic effects such as growth and maturation of long bones

fatty acid: an organic compound composed of carbon, hydrogen, and oxygen; combines with glycerol to form fat; one of the by-products of the metabolism of fat

free radical: an atom or molecule with an impaired electron; produced in the course of normal metabolism, in the breakdown of oxidized fats in the body, by radiation, and by stress

gastritis: inflammation of the lining of the stomach

genetic blueprint: the body chemistry you inherited from your parents

genetic potential: inherited potential genetic blueprint

gland: an organ which manufactures a chemical which will be utilized elsewhere; if this chemical secretion goes into the bloodstream, the gland belongs to the endocrine system; if the chemical secretes through a duct (tube) to surrounding tissues, it is an exocrine gland

glucose: a simple sugar, also called dextrose or grape sugar, found in fruits, vegetables, the sap of trees, honey, corn syrup, and molasses; the end product of the digestion of starch, sucrose, maltose, and lactose, it provides most of the energy for the cells of the body

glycogen: the main form of carbohydrate stored in the liver and muscles

glyconeogenesis: glycogen synthesized by the liver from fats and proteins

gonad: sex gland; the ovary or testicle

hemoglobin: the pigment in the red blood cells, it is the substance which carries oxygen to the tissue

high-density lipoprotein: fraction of the blood containing fats and proteins; associated with a reduced risk in heart disease

homeopathy: a branch of medicine characterized by treatment of illness with small doses of drugs that produce, in a healthy person, symptoms like those of the illness being treated

homeostasis (homeostatic mechanism): a mechanism used by the body to maintain a stable chemical internal environment, despite external change; this is accomplished in large part by the hormones

hormone: a chemical produced by a gland, secreted into the blood, and affecting the function of distant cells or organs

hydrochloric acid: hydrogen chloride, an acid secreted by the cells lining the stomach which is helpful in the digestion of food

hyper-: prefix meaning "excessive," "above"

hyperglycemia: diabetes (mellitus)

hypoglycemia: too little sugar in the blood

hypothalamus: the master gland of the neuroendocrine system; controls the brain, the pituitary's production, and the release of its own hormone

immune complex: antigen combined with antibody; tissue damage is caused when the complexes are formed in the presence of complement and leukocytes

immunoglobulins: a family of plasma protein to which the antibodies belong; subdivided into five classes: IgG, IgA, IgE, IgM, and IgF (Ig stands for immunoglobulin)

inflammation: a process consisting of reactions that occur in the affected blood vessels and adjacent tissues in response to an injury or abnormal stimulation caused by physical, chemical, or biological agent(s); characterized by swelling, pain, increased temperature, and redness in the region of injury due to increased local blood flow

insulin: a hormone produced in the islets of Langerhans of the pancreas; when secreted into the bloodstream, it permits the metabolism and utilization of sugar

islets of Langerhans: the cells in the pancreas that secrete insulin

leukocyte: white blood cell

lipid: fat

low-density lipoprotein: fraction of blood containing fats and proteins; associated with an increase in heart disease

menopause: the change of life; the time of life when a woman's menstrual period ceases

metabolic rate: the rate at which food is broken down in the body

metabolism: the process by which foods are transformed into basic elements which can be utilized by the body for energy or growth

mineral: any chemical compound found in nature and not containing carbon

naturopath: a practitioner who used foods, supplements, water, and light in treatment of illness

orthomolecular doctor: one who treats infectious and degenerative diseases by varying the concentration of substances such as vitamins, minerals, trace elements, amino acids, enzymes, essential fatty acids, and hormones which are normally present in the human body

osteoarthritis: a form of arthritis associated with bone and cartilage degeneration

osteoporosis: loss of bone or skeletal tissue, producing brittleness or softness of bone

pancreas: a gland in upper portion of the abdomen which secretes the hormones insulin and glucagon into bloodstream, and secretes digestive enzymes and bicarbonate into the intestine

parathyroid gland: one of four small endocrine glands located in the neck; secretes the hormone which controls calcium and phosphorus metabolism

pepsin: an enzyme secreted into the intestinal tract to aid in the digestion of food, particularly protein

periodontal disease: a disease of the tissues, including the gums, immediately surrounding the teeth (pyorrhea)

pH: a symbol denoting acidity or alkalinity

phagocyte: white blood cell which can eat or destroy foreign matter or bacteria

pituitary: an endocrine gland in the base of the brain; secretes several hormones and seems to control the secretions of other glands such as the thyroid and adrenals

polypeptides: intermediate state of the breakdown of protein; can do harm if they enter the bloodstream before broken down into amino acids

postpituitary gland (posterior pituitary): a portion of the pituitary which secretes hormones such as an antidiuretic hormone

postprandial: following a meal

progesterone: a steroid hormone secreted primarily by ovaries and placenta; stimulates secretion by uterine glands, inhibits contraction of uterine smooth muscle, and stimulates breast growth

prostaglandins: a group of fatty acids which function as chemical messengers, made in most, possibly all, cells of the body; transmit chemical signals between cells or between one area of a cell and another area

rarefy: to make or become thin or less dense

rheumatoid arthritis: joint inflammation, often affecting many joints simultaneously; characterized by pain and limitation of motion

sodium bicarbonate: a mild alkali secreted by the pancreas or may be taken by mouth; used extensively to neutralize excess stomach acid; used to counteract an allergic reaction

thyroid: endocrine gland located in front of the neck; regulates body metabolism; secretes a hormone known as thyroxin

thyroxin: the hormone manufactured by the thyroid gland

triglycerides: a class of fat found in the bloodstream

victim: not known in this book

Bibliography

Many of the references used in this bibliography were jotted down long before thoughts of publishing a book occurred. As a result, the listings of some of these references are incomplete, but are included here in hopes that they will nonetheless be a help to the reader.

Chapter 1. I Was a Sugarholic
Coca, Arthur F., M.D. *The Pulse Test*. New York: Arco Publishing Company, 1978.

Chapter 2. Sugar's Unbalancing Act
Bland, Jeffrey, Ph.D. *Digestive Enzymes*. New Canaan, Conn.: Keats Publishing, 1983.

Frame, Boy, M.D., and Geoffrey Marel, M.D., "Reflections on Bone Disease in Total Parenteral Nutrition." In *Metabolic Bone Disease in Total Parenteral Nutrition*. Edited by Jack W. Coburn, M.D., and Gordon L. Klein, M.D. Baltimore: Urban and Schwarzenberg, 1985.

Page, Melvin, D.D.S. *Body Chemistry in Health and Disease*. Reprinted by Price-Pottenger Nutrition Foundation, La Mesa, Calif.

Page, Melvin, D.D.S., and H. Leon Abram, Jr. *Your Body Is Your Best Doctor*. New Canaan, Conn.: Keats Publishing, 1972.

Randolph, Theron, M.D., and Leona B. Yeager, M.D. "Corn Sugar as an Allergen." *Annals of Allergy*, Sept.–Oct. 1949, 650–61.

Wade, Carlson. *Helping Your Health with Enzymes*. New York: ARC Books, 1971.

Chapter 3. All About Allergies
Bjeldanes, Leonard. "Effect of Over-Cooked Meat." *Journal of Food and Chemical Toxicology* 23, no. 12 (April 1985).

Brown, H. Harrow, M.D. "The Diagnosis and Management of Allergy." Paper delivered at the annual meeting of the Indian College of Allergy and Immunology, Simla, Ariz., Sept. 1980.

Hills, Amelia Nathan. Amelia Nathan Hill International Foundation of Collating Allergy Research, Wimbledon, England, Apr. 4, 1983. Personal interview.

Kaslow, Arthur L., M.D., and Richard B. Miles. *Freedom from Chronic Disease*. Los Angeles: J. P. Tarcher, 1979.

Rea, William, M.D., et al. "Food and Chemical Susceptibility After Environmental Chemical Overexposure: Case Histories." *Annals of Allergy* 41 (August 1978): 101–10.

Ulett, George A., M.D. "Food Allergy—Cytotoxic Testing and the Central Nervous System." *Psychiatric Journal of the University of Ottawa* 5, no. 2 (June 1980).

Wallach, Joel. "Metabolic Therapy." Paper delivered at the National Health Federation Meeting, Long Beach, Calif. Jan. 1983. Tape.

Willeke, K., and K. Whitley. "Aerosols: Size Distribution Interpretation." *Air Pollution Control Association Journal* 25, no. 526: 196.

Chapter 4. The Destruction of the Immune System
Dufty, William. *Sugar Blues*. New York: Warner Books, 1975.

Kijak, Ernest, D.D.S., George Foust, D.D.S., and Ralph Steinman, D.D.S., M.S. "Relationship of Blood Sugar Level and Leukocytic Phagocytosis." *Southern California State Dental Association Journal* 32, no. 9 (Sept. 1964).

Philpott, William H., M.D., and Dwight K. Kalita, Ph.D. *Brain Allergies*. New Canaan, Conn.: Keats Publishing, 1980.

Sanchez, A., et al. "Role of Sugars in Human Neutrophilic Phagocytosis." *American Journal of Clinical Nutrition*. Nov. 1973, 1180–84.

Selye, Hans, M.D. *The Stress of Life*. San Francisco: McGraw-Hill, 1978.

Chapter 5. The Consequences
Ulett, George, M.D., Ph.D. "Food Allergy—Cytotoxic Testing and the Central Nervous System." *Psychiatric Journal of the University of Ottawa* 5, no. 2 (June 1980): 100–108

HYPOGLYCEMIA
Smith, Lendon, M.D., *Feed Yourself Right*. New York: Dell Publishing Co., Inc., 1983.

DIABETES
Brekhman, I. I., and I. F. Nesterenko. *Brown Sugar and Health*. New York: Pergamon Press, 1983.

Philpott, William H., M.D., and Dwight K. Kalita, Ph.D. *Victory over Diabetes*. New Canaan, Conn.: Keats Publishing, 1983.

Saner, G. "Urinary Chromium Excretion During Pregnancy and Relationship with Intravenous Glucose Loading." *American Journal of Clinical Nutrition* 34 (1981): 1676.

Shannon, Ira L., D.M.D., M.S.D. *Brand Name Guide to Sugar*. Chicago: Nelson Hall, 1977.

ARTHRITIS

Buckley, Rebecca, M.D. "Food Allergy." *Journal of the American Medical Association* 248 (1982): 2627.

Catterall, William E. "Rheumatoid Arthritis Is an Allergy." *Arthritis News Today*, 1980.

Darlington, L. G., N. W. Ramsey, and J. R. Mansfield. "Placebo-Controlled, Blind Study of Dietary Manipulatio. Therapy in Rheumatoid Arthritis." *Lancet*, Feb. 6, 1986, 236–38.

Wiggins, Roger C., M.R.C.P., and M. P. Cochrane. "Immune Complex—Medicated Biological Effects." *New England Journal of Medicine* 304 (1981): 518.

ASTHMA

Gaby, Alan R., M.D. *The Doctor's Guide to Vitamin B_6*. Emmaus, Pa.: Rodale Press, 1983.

Power, Lawrence, M.D. "Sensitivity: You React to What You Eat." *Los Angeles Times*, Feb. 12, 1985.

HEADACHES

Egger, J., et al. "Is Migraine Food Allergy?" *Lancet*, Oct. 15, 1983, 865–67.

Grant, Ellen, M.D. "Food Allergy and Migraine." *Lancet* 8123 (1979): 966–69.

Power, Lawrence, M.D. "Special Diets Ease Some Headache Pain." *Los Angeles Times*, Aug. 12, 1984.

Tauroso, Nicola Michael, M.D., F.A.A.P. "Allergy and Sensitivities." *Living Health Bulletin* 2 (1984): 13–149.

PSORIASIS

Douglass, John M., M.D., Internal Medicine, and coordinator of the Health Improvement Service, Southern California, Kaiser Medical Group, Los Angeles. "Psoriasis and Diet." *Western Journal of Medicine* 133 (Nov. 1980): 450.

OSTEOPOROSIS

Notelovitz, Morris, M.D., and Marsha Ware. *Stand Tall: Every Woman's Guide to Preventing Osteoporosis*. New York: Bantam Books, 1985.

"Osteoporosis in Young Men." *Healthwise* 6, no. 1 (Jan. 1983).

Poulos, Jean, Ph.D. "The Nutritional Approach to Osteoporosis." *Nutritional Consultant*, Feb. 1984, 25.

CANCER

LeShan, Lawrence. *You Can Fight for Your Life*. New York: Evans Publishing Co., 1980.

Warberg, Otto, M.D. *The Metabolism of Tumours*. London: Constable & Co., 1930.

CANDIDA ALBICANS

Crook, William G., M.D. *The Yeast Connection*. Jackson, Tenn.: Professional Books, 1984.

Rose Elizabeth. *Lady of Gray*. Santa Monica, Calif.: Butterfly Publishing Co., 1985.

Lorenzani, Shirley, Ph.D. "Candida Albicans." Cassette tapes, set I and II. La Mesa, Calif.: Price-Pottenger Nutrition Foundation, 1978.

Truss, C. Orion, M.D. *The Missing Diagnosis*. Birmingham, Ala., 1983. P.O. Box 26508, Birmingham, Ala. 35226.

————. "Restoration of Immunologic Competence to Candida Albicans." *Orthomolecular Psychiatry* 9, no. 4, 1980: 287–301.

HEART DISEASE
Brekhman, I. I., and I. F. Nesterenko. *Brown Sugar and Health*. New York: Pergamon Press, 1983.

Doisy, R. J. *Minerals and Trace Elements*, pp. 586–94. (Publisher unknown.)

Goulart, Frances Sheridan. "Behind Bars, Kicking the Candy Bar Habit." Parts 1, 2. *Herbalist New Health*, Jan., Feb., 1981.

Hallfrisch, J., et al. "The Effects of Fructose on Blood Lipid Levels." *American Journal of Clinical Nutrition* 37, no. 5 (1983): 740–48.

McKenzie, M. M. "Urinary Excretion of Cadmium, Zinc and Copper in Hypertensive Women." *New England Medical Journal* 80, 68–70.

Philpott, William H., M.D., and Dwight K. Kalita, Ph.D. *Victory over Diabetes*. New Canaan, Conn.: Keats Publishing, 1983.

Raboff, J. "Oxidized Lipids: A Key to Heart Disease." *Science News* 129:278.

Robinson, Miles H., M.D., "On Sugar and White Flour— the Dangerous Twins." In *A Physician's Handbook to Orthomolecular Medicine*. Edited by Roger William, M.D., and Dwight K. Kalita. New York: Pergamon Press, 1978. Pp. 24–28.

Wolf, R. N., and S. M. Grundy. "Influence of Exchanging Carbohydrate for Saturated Fatty Acids on Plasma Lipids and Lipoproteins in Men." *Journal of Nutrition* 113 (1983): 1521.

Yudkin, John, M.D. "Dietary Fat and Dietary Sugar in Relation to Ischemic Heart Disease and Diabetes." *Lancet* 2, no. 4 (1964).

————. *Sweet and Dangerous*. New York: Bantam Books, 1972.

TOOTH DECAY
Ashmead, DeWayne, Ph.D. *Chelated Mineral Nutrition*. Huntington Beach, Calif. Institute Publishers, 1981.

Steinman, Ralph, D.D.S. Loma Linda University research on the effects of sugar on tooth decay. Information not published. Private communication via Bruce Pacetti, D.D.S.

Wilson, Eva D., Katherine H. Fisher, and Pilar A. Garcia. *Principles of Nutrition*. New York: John Wiley & Sons, 1979.

MULTIPLE SCLEROSIS
Erlander, Stig R., Ph.D. "The Cause and Cure of Multiple Sclerosis." *The Diet to End Disease* 1, no. 3 (Mar. 3, 1979): 59–63.

Kaslow, Arthur L., M.D., and Richard B. Miles. *Freedom from Chronic Disease*. Los Angeles: J. P. Tarcher, 1979.

Lazarus, Pat. "Multiple Sclerosis and Amyotrophic Lateral Sclerosis: More Hope Than We Think." *Let's Live*, Apr. 1980, 70–77.

Liversidge, L. A. "Treatment and Management of Multiple Sclerosis." *British Medical Bulletin* 33 (1977): 78–83.

Null, Gary. "A Trio of Distinguished Doctors Discuss Successful MS Treatment." *Bestways*, Oct. 1981, 35–40, 125.

Zucker, Martin. "Fight Back! Don't Learn to Live with M.S." *Let's Live*, Dec. 1982, 10–14.

INFLAMMATORY BOWEL DISEASE
Galton, Lawrence. *You May Not Need a Psychiatrist*. New York: Simon & Schuster, 1979.

Garmon, Linda. "Crohn's Disease: Intestinal Enigma." *Science News* 177 (May 3, 1980): 280–81.

Jones, V. A., et al. "Food Intolerance: A Major Factor in the Pathogenesis of Irritable Bowel Syndrome." *Lancet*, Nov. 10, 1982, 1115–17.

Jones, V. A., et al. "Crohn's Disease: Maintenance of Remission by Diet." *Lancet*, July 27, 1985, 177–80.

Pearson, D. J., K. Rix and S. Bently. "Food Allergy, How Much in the Mind." *Lancet* 2 (1983): 1259–61.

Petitpierre, M., P. Guimowski, and J. P. Girard. "Irritable Bowel Syndrome and Hypersensitivity to Food." *Annals of Allergy* 54 (June 1985): 538–40.

CANKER SORES
Power, Lawrence. "Change in Diet May Help Relieve Asthma Patient." *Los Angeles Times*, May 7, 1985.

GALLSTONES
Challem, Jack Joseph and Renate Lewin. "Vitamins and Fiber for Preventing Gallstones." *Let's Live*, April 14, 1984, 10–12.

Heaton K. W. "The Sweet Road to Gallstones." *British Medical Journal* 288 (Apr. 14, 1984): 1103–4.

CYSTIC FIBROSIS
Braganza, J. M. "Selenium Deficiency, Cystic Fibrosis, and Pancreatic Cancer." *Lancet* 2 (1986): 1238.

Stead, R. J., et al. "Selenium Deficiency and Possible Increased Risk of Carcinoma in Adults with Cystic Fibrosis." *Lancet* 2 (1986): 862.

Wallach, J. D., and B. Germaise. "Cystic Fibrosis: A Perinatal Manifestation of Selenium Deficiency." *Trace Sub-*

stances in Environmental Health. Edited by D. D. Hemphill. Columbia, Mo.: University of Missouri Press, 1979.

FUTURE GENERATIONS
Pottenger, Francis M., Jr., M.D. *Pottenger's Cats*. La Mesa, Calif.: Price-Pottenger Nutrition Foundation, 1983.

Ulett, George A., M.D. "Food Allergy—Cytotoxic Testing and the Central Nervous System." *Psychiatric Journal of the University of Ottawa* 5, no. 2 (June, 1980): 100–108.

Wallach, Joel. "Metabolic Therapy for Heart Disease, Cancer, Allergies and Multiple Sclerosis." Paper presented at the National Health Federation, Long Beach, Calif., Jan. 1983. Tape.

Chapter 6. Sugar's Helpers
ALCOHOL
Adams, Ruth, and Frank Murray. *Megavitamin Therapy*. New York: Larchmont Books, 1973.

Ashmead, DeWayne, Ph.D. *Chelated Mineral Nutrition*. Huntington Beach, Calif.: Institute Publishers, 1981.

Bjarnason, Ingvar, Kevin Ward, and Timothy Peters. "The Leaky Gut of Alcoholism: Possible Route of Entry for Toxic Compounds." *Lancet* 8370 (Jan. 28, 1984).

Davenport, H. W. "Why the Stomach Does Not Digest Itself." *Scientific American* 226 (Jan. 1972): 87–93.

Philpott, William, M.D., and Dwight K. Kalita, Ph.D. *Victory over Diabetes*. New Canaan, Conn.: Keats Publishing, 1983.

Randolph, Theron G., M.D. "Is Allergy the Root of Alcoholism?" *Bestways*, Mar. 1983, 44–49.

Randolph, Theron G., M.D., and Ralph W. Moss, Ph.D. *An Alternative Approach to Allergies*. New York: Bantam Books, 1981.

Smith, Lendon H., M.D. *Improving Your Child's Behavior Chemistry*. New York: Pocket Books, 1976.

Ulett, George A., M.D. "Food Allergy—Cytotoxic Testing and the Central Nervous System." *Psychiatric Journal of the University of Ottawa* 5, no. 2 (June, 1980) 100–108.

Zucher, Martin. "Nutrition and the Addicted." *Let's Live,* June 1980, 16.

CAFFEINE

Bland, Jeffrey, Ph.D. *Your Health Under Siege*. Brattleboro, Vt.: The Stephen Green Press, 1981.

Ritter, E. J., et al. "Potentiative Interaction Between Caffeine and Various Teratogenic Agents." *Teratology* 25, no. 95 (1982).

Wallis, Claudia. "Stress—Can We Cope?" *Time*, June 6, 1983, 48–54.

ASPIRIN

Bennett, William, M.D. Oregon Health Science University, Portland, Oregon. Personal interview, June 10, 1986.

Cimons, Marlene. "New Study Strongly Links Aspirin, Reye's Syndrome." *Los Angeles Times*, Feb. 1, 1985.

Davenport, H. W. "Why The Stomach Does Not Digest Itself." *Scientific American* 226 (Jan. 1972): 87–93.

Dufty, William. *Sugar Blues*. New York: Warner Books, 1975.

Klenner, Frederick Robert. "Significance of High Daily Intake of Ascorbic Acid in Preventive Medicine." In *A Physician's Handbook to Orthomolecular Medicine*. Edited by Roger Williams, M.D., and Dwight K. Kalita. New York: Pergamon Press, 1978.

Levine, Stephen. "Oxidants and Antioxidants and Chemical Sensitivities." *Allergy Research Review* 2, no.1 (Spring 1981).

Muther, Richard S., M.D., Donald M. Potter, M.D., and William Bennett, M.D. "Aspirin-Induced Depression of Glomerular Filtration Rate in Normal Humans: Role of Sodium Balance." *Annals of Internal Medicine* 94 (1981): 317–21.

Prescott, L. F. "Analgesic Nephropathy." *Drugs* 23 (1982): 75–149.

Stanley, Edith, M.D., et al. "Increased Virus Shedding with Aspirin Treatment of Rhinovirus Infection." *Journal of the American Medical Association*, Mar. 24, 1975.

Vander, Arthur, M.D., James Sherman, Ph.D., and Dorothy Luciano, Ph.D. *Human Physiology*. New York: McGraw-Hill Publishing, 1980.

DRUGS

Joas, C., H. Kewitz, and D. Reenhold-Kouniati. "Effects of Diuretics of Plasma Lipoproteins in Healthy Men." *European Journal of Clinical Pharmacology* 17 (1980): 251–57.

Spencer, Herta, M.D., and Lois Kramer, R.D. "Antacids-Induced Calcium Loss." *Archives of Internal Medicine* 143, no.4 (1983): 657–58

Widell, Elna. "Those Allergenic Sweet Nothings in Your Pharmaceutical Pill." *Environmental Illness Association Newsletter*, July 1984. C/o Barri Boone, 2417 Ivy Drive, #3, Oakland, CA 94606.

RANCID FATS

Bjeldanes, Leonard. "Effects of High Temperatures on Meats." *Food and Chemical Toxicology* 23, no.12 (Apr. 1985).

Pariza, Michael W., Ph.D. *Diet and Cancer*. Summit, N. J.: American Council on Science and Health, 1985.

Lyinsky, W., and P. Shuber. "Benzo-Pyrene and Other Polynuclear Hydrocarbons in Charbroiled Meat." *Science* 145:2 (1985).

OTHER OVERCOOKED FOOD
Pottenger, Francis M., Jr., M.D. *Pottenger's Cats*. LaMesa, Calif.: Price Pottenger Nutritional Foundation, 1983.

FOOD ADDITIVES
Abrahams, Cyril, M.D., Koshilya Rijhsinghani, M.D., and Martin Swerdlow. "Tumor Induction in Mice Following Administration of DEA-HCl and $NaNO_2$." *Cancer Detection and Prevention* 5, no. 3 (1982): 283–90.

Hunter, Beatrice Trum. *Food Additives and Your Health*. New Canaan, Conn.: Keats Publishing, 1972.

Mayron, Lewis W., and Erwin Kaplan, M.D. "The Use of Chronium—51 Sodium Chromate for the Detection of Food and Chemical Sensitivities." *Annals of Allergy* 38 (1977): 323.

SWEETENERS
Carroll, Lewis. *Alice's Adventures in Wonderland* and *Through the Looking Glass*. New York: Bantam Books, 1981.

Shurkin, Joel N. "Artificial Sweeteners." *Healthline*, Oct. 1983, 10.

"Sugar Substitutes." *Medical Hotline* 4, no.4 (Apr.–May 1983): 1. New York: Medical News Associates.

MERCURY
Ashmead, DeWayne, Ph.D. *Chelated Mineral Nutrition*. Huntington Beach, Calif.: Institute Publishers, 1981.

Kupsinel, Roy, M.D. "A Patient's Guide to Mercury Amalgam Toxicity." Oviedo, Fla.: Keeps Komments, 1984.

Ziff, Sam. *The Toxic Time Bomb*. New York: Aurora Press, 1984.

Chapter 7. Stress

Brekhman, I. I., and I. F. Nesterenko. *Brown Sugar and Health*. New York: Pergamon Press, 1983.

Linn, Margaret, et al. Veterans Administration Medical Center, Miami, Fla. Cited in American Institute for Cancer Research Information Sheet, 1985.

Selye, Hans, M.D. *Stress Without Distress*. New York: Signet, 1974.

————. *The Stress of Life*. New York: McGraw-Hill Book Co., 1976.

Schleifer, Steven, et al. "A Simplified Method for Assaying PHA Induced Stimulation of Rat Peripheral Blood Lymphocytes." *Journal of Immunological Methods* 51, no. 3 (1982): 287–91.

Chapter 8. A Practical Life Plan for Attaining and Maintaining Good Health

Pacetti, Bruce, D.D.S., and Nancy Appleton, Ph.D. *How to Monitor Your Basic Health*. Santa Monica, Calif.: Choice Publishing Co., 1985.

Schneider, Keith. " 'Miracle Cure'—Holism or Hokum?" *New Age*, Sept., 1985, 12.

Shames, Richard L., M.D. "About Aids." *Holistic Health* (Nov. 1985): 26–28.

Reference Books and Articles on Sugar

Abrahamson, E. M., M.D., and A. W. Pezet. *Body, Mind and Sugar*. New York: Avon Books, 1951.

Brekhman, I. I., and I. F. Nesterenko. *Brown Sugar and Health*. New York: Pergamon Press, 1983.

Cannon, G. "The Sugar Lobby." *Lancet*, Jan. 26, 1985.

Cheraskin, E., M.D., D.M.D., and W. M. Ringsdorf, Jr., D.M.D., M.S., with Arline Brecher. *Psychodietetics*. New York: Bantam Books, 1978.

Cleave, T. L. *The Saccharine Disease*. New Canaan, Conn.: Keats Publishing, 1974.

Cleave, T. L., and G. D. Campbell. *Diabetes, Coronary Thrombosis and the Saccharine Disease*. Bristol, England: John Wright & Sons, 1969.

Deerr, N. *The History of Sugar*. London: Chapman & Hall Co., 1949.

Dufty, William. *Sugar Blues*. New York: Warner Books, 1975.

Gerstenzang, Sharon D. *Cook with Me Sugar Free*. New York: Simon & Schuster, 1983.

Hunter, Beatrice Trum. *The Sugar Primer*. Charlotte, N.C.: Garden Way Publishing, 1979.

————. *The Sugar Trap and How to Avoid It*. Boston: Houghton Mifflin Co., 1982.

Jenkins, David, et al. "Glycemic Index of Foods: A Physiological Basis for Carbohydrate Exchange." *American Journal of Clinical Nutrition* 34:360–66.

Rogers, S. "Sugar and Health." *Lancet*, Feb. 23, 1985.

Schauss, Alexander. *Diet, Crime and Delinquency*. Berkeley, Calif.: Parker House, 1981.

Shannon, Ira L. *Brand Name Guide to Sugar*. Chicago: Nelson Hall, 1977.

Wilson, David. *Sugar and Food Additives*. Black Mountain, N.C.: Loren House.

Yudkin, John, M.D. "Sugar and Disease." *Nature* 239:197–99.

————. "Sugar for Debate." *Lancet*, Mar. 30, 1985.

————. *Sweet and Dangerous*. New York: Bantam Books, 1972.

INDEX

acidosis, 35
acute reaction, 32–33
Adams, Ruth, 81
adaption, 30, 32, 34–35
alcohol, 78–81
Alcoholics Anonymous (AA), 79–80
allergies:
    in babies, 23–24, 32, 33
    brain, 35
    food, 3–4, 10, 21–26, 31
    inhalant, 26–27
allergy addiction, 34
Appleton, Nancy, 10
arthritis, 42, 49–50
Ashmead, DeWayne, 95
aspirin, 89–91
asthma, 42, 51–52

Biological Stress Syndrome, 30
Bland, Jeffrey, 82
bohemian spiced tomato soup, 129
Brekhman, I. I., 100
British Medical Journal, 73
broccoli and potatoes vinaigrette, 137
broccoli soup with vegetables, 128–129
Bulgarian bean salad, 135

cabbage scramble, 133
caffeine, 34, 35, 81–83
calcium-urine test, 48, 49, 109–110
cancer, 42, 54–56
candida albicans, 42, 67–68
canker sores, 42, 73
Catterall, William, 50
chronic reaction, 33–35
Chron's disease, 71
Coca, Arthur, F., 3–4

constipation, 42, 46–48
Cook, James, D., 82
curried peppers and garbanzos, 131
cystic fibrosis, 42, 74
cytotoxic reactions, 37
cytotoxic tests, 52

degenerative disease process, 7–8, 30
    stages of, 31–37
degenerative reaction, 36–37
diabetes, 39, 42, 44–46
Doisy, R. J., 63–64
Douglass, John M., 53
drugs, 83–86
Dunaif, George, 88

endocrine glands, 17–19
enzymes, 19–20, 31
exhaustion, 30, 32, 36

food additives, 91–92
food allergies, 3–4, 10, 21–27, 31, 34
Food and Drug Administration (FDA), 82, 93
    94
food categories, 112–116
food plans, 110–111
fresh potato melange, 130

gallstones, 42, 73–74
garbure, 126
General Adaption Syndrome, 30–31
genetic blueprints, 36, 37, 55, 74, 108
gingery chicken soup, 127

Hallfrisch, J., 64
headaches, 42, 52–53
    see also migraines

159

health maintenance, 103–104
  arenas of, 105–109
health-promoting eating habits, 117
heart disease, 42, 62–65
hearty beet borscht, 129
hot asparagus soup, 127
hot borscht, 130
hypoglycemia, 42–44, 119

inflammatory bowel disease, 42, 71–72
immune systems, destruction of, 30–40
intestinal gass, 42, 48–49
Irish stew, 133
islets of Langerhans, 42, 44

joint pains, 31, 33
  see also arthritis

Kaslow, Arthur, 71
Kummerow, Fred A., 63

lentil tomato loaf, 133
LeShan, Lawrence, 99
Linn, Margaret, 99
Loma Linda University, 37–40, 70

McKenzie, M. M., 64
Manhattan clam chowder, Mexican style, 128
Marel, Geoffrey, 15
mayonnaise, basic, 136
Mayron, Lewis, 91
meat dishes, 133–135
mercury, 95–96
migraines, 33
minerals, 15–16, 31, 44
molded chicken salad, 136
monosodium glutamate (MSG), 52
Monte, Woodrow C., 94
multiple sclerosis (MS), 42, 71

National Toxicology Program, 83
NutraSweet, 93, 121

obesity, 42, 65–67
osteoporosis, 42, 56–61
overcooked food, 87–89

Pacetti, Bruce, 110
Page, Melvin, 13–14
pepper slaw, 137
peppers stuffed with barley and corn, 130–131
Persian lamb and bean stew with herbs, 134–135
Philpott, William H., 62, 64, 79

Pottenger, Francis, 75, 88
Potts, John, 45
psoriasis, 42, 53
psychological stress, sugar and, 99–101
Pulse Test, The (Coca), 3

rancid fats, 86–87
Randolph, Theron, 23
ratatouille, 132
Rea, William J., 27
required daily allowance (RDA), 13
Reye's syndrome, 90–91

saccharin, 94, 121
salad dressings, 135–137
salads, 135–137
savory pepper pilaf, 131–132
Schleifer, Steven, 99
Schneeman, Barbara, 88
Selye, Hans, 30, 32, 63
Senate Dietary Goals, 65
Simonton Visualization Method, 109
soups, 126–130
Spanish-style rice and ground beef, 134
Stanley, Edith, 89, 90
Steinman, Ralph, 70
stress, 97
  how to handle, 101–102
  psychological, 98–99
Stress Without Distress (Selye), 30
sugarholics, 1–5, 10
  self-help techniques for, 118–123
  tests for, 5–7
sweeteners, 93–95, 121

Takaahushi, Eyi, 83
tooth decay, 42, 68–71
Truss, C. Orin, 67

Ulett, George, 23, 79

vegetable chowder, 128
vegetable rice salad, 136
vegetables, 130–133
vegetarian stew, 132

Walberg, Otto, 54
Wallach, Joel, 24, 74
Wayne, John, 55–56
Wurtman, Richard, 94

Yudkin, John, 62, 85

AUDIO CASSETTES

An extensive look at each of these subjects is available on tape cassettes.

LICK THE SUGAR HABIT—This tape is an introduction to the book. It explains, in detail, the body chemistry principle, mineral relationships, the endocrine system, enzymes, and what promotes infectious and degenerative diseases. (1 hour)

ALLERGIES—The subjects of this tape are allergies, what causes them, and how to eliminate them. Learn how foods to which you react can be reintroduced back into your diet. The subject of inhalant allergies is also explored. (1 hour)

OSTEOPOROSIS—You may be getting a reasonable amount of calcium in your diet, but, if you are eating abusive foods or upsetting your life-style in other ways, the calcium will not absorb as well. What you do not eat is more important than what you do eat. This tape tells how to look for symptoms and how to test for susceptibility to osteoporosis. (1 hour)

OBESITY—The newest research on what works and what doesn't is discussed. You will understand the relationship of allergies, addictions and cravings to obesity. (1/2 hour) WOMEN/opposite side.

WOMEN—Premenstrual syndrome (P.M.S.), Candida Albicans (yeast infections), menses, menopause, and post menopausal problems are discussed on this tape. (1/2 hour) OBESITY/opposite side.

CHILDREN—The first subject on this tape is nutrition during pregnancy. Infants' and children's eating problems are then discussed, as well as children's allergies. Ideas to help teenagers eat nutritious foods end the tape. (1 hour)

FOOD PREPARATION—Where and how to buy food, insecticides, fungicides, food irradiation, additives, vitamins, minerals, and how to prepare food so that it will not upset the body chemistry are discussed. (1 hour)

URINE AND PH TESTING—Information is given as to how to test for homeostasis of urine and saliva. Suggestions are given as to what causes upset body chemistry and how to help balance it. (1 hour)

NEW INFORMATION—Information from medical journals linking health, the medical field, and nutrition. (1 hour)

	One*	Two*	Three*	Four*
Price of tape	$ 6.00	$12.00	$15.00	$20.00
Sales Tax (Calif. only)	$ .50	$ .99	$ 1.24	$ 1.65
Shipping	$ 1.00	$ 1.25	$ 1.50	$ 1.75

	Five*	Six*	Seven*	Eight*
Price of tape	$25.00	$30.00	$35.00	$40.00
Sales Tax (Calif. only)	$ 2.06	$ 2.48	$ 2.89	$ 2.99
Shipping	$ 2.00	$ 2.00	$ 2.00	$ 2.00

*Specify which tape(s) you want. Make check payable to:

Nancy Appleton, Ph.D.
P.O. Box 3083
Santa Monica, CA 90403

ORDER FORM
BODY CHEMISTRY TEST KIT

This kit is used to determine if your minerals are in the correct relationship to each other and if your body chemistry is in balance. The kit includes solution to use for 250 tests, two test tubes, an eye dropper, a brush for cleaning test tubes, and the instruction book, *Monitoring Your Basic Health*. The book contains a section on what upsets body chemistry, suggestions on how to balance body chemistry, food plans, and a section on how to test for food allergies. pH paper to test for acid-alkalinity of the saliva is also included.

NAME: _____

ADDRESS: _____ APT: _____

CITY: _____

STATE: _____ ZIP: _____

1 kit	$20.00
Shipping	$ 1.50
Sales tax (California residents only)	$ 1.65

Make check payable to:

Nancy Appleton, Ph.D.
P.O. Box 3083
Santa Monica, CA 90403-3083